Nuclear Survival Guide

Essential Tactics and Strategies for Immediate Family Safety

(Life Saving Nuclear Facts Self-help Instructions and Skills for Surviving Nuclear War)

Edward Lopez

Published By **Simon Dough**

Edward Lopez

Nuclear Survival Guide: Essential Tactics and Strategies for Immediate Family Safety (Life Saving Nuclear Facts Self-help Instructions and Skills for Surviving Nuclear War)

ISBN   978-1-9994868-3-9

Legal & Disclaimer

Table Of Contents

Chapter 1: Nuclear War Survival Skills Manual

Fundamentals

Nuclear bombs are among the most deadly weapons available on the globe. They are powered by releases of energy via nuclear fusion or nuclear fission. The energy released is through radiation and heat, which may cause irreparable damages to the infrastructure as well as people.

Nuclear bombs are generally classed by yield which is the quantity of energy released. The biggest nuclear weapon that has ever used was that of in the Soviet Union's "Tsar Bomba" that had the yield of 50 megatons, which is the equivalent of more than three thousand Hiroshima-sized nuclear weapons.

"Tsar Bomba" was massive enough that it caused destruction to people and the surrounding environment that lived 62 miles from the location of the explosion. The consequences of a nuclear weapon are influenced by a variety of variables, such as the power of the weapon as well as the elevation where it's detonated along with weather conditions, as well as the kind of terrain in which the explosion occurs.

But, generally speaking, nuclear bombs could cause massive destruction and cause death. They are regarded as among the most deadly weapons currently that exist and are strictly restricted under the international laws.

But, given recent news regarding the conflict in Ukraine The parties involved have been contemplating the use of strategic nuclear bombs, in spite of the limitations that are imposed in international laws. Therefore, it's important to know the consequences of using it and to prepare for the worst-case situation.

How do nuclear bombs function

What is the process of making nuclear bombs? Simply put the nuclear bombs function with the help of nuclear fission in order to produce the possibility of an explosion. Nuclear fission involves the method of breaking atoms in the event that it is employed to make a bomb, it is able to create a explosive explosion.

Nuclear bombs consist of two components which are: the nuclear fuel and the detonator. The fuel used in nuclear bombs is typically plutonium or uranium and it's the latter that is subject to fission after the bomb explodes. Detonators are what set off the fission process which can take place with anything from an electrical charge or a complicated chemical reaction.

If the detonator is activated this triggers the chain reaction that produces nuclear fission. These reaction releases an enormous quantity of energy which causes the explosive. The intensity of the explosion will depend on the quantity of nuclear fuel utilized. The more fuel used, the greater the blast.

It's crucial to understand that nuclear weapons aren't simply big firecrackers, they're extremely deadly weapons. The explosion from a nuclear weapon can destroy entire towns, and the radiation emitted can be a serious health risk when exposed to the radiation. Nuclear weapons should not be taken lightly and their destructive power shouldn't be overlooked.

Different types of nuclear bombs

Three kinds of weapons that are associated with the notion of nuclear bombs.

*The Atomic Bomb: leverages a fission reaction.

The thermonuclear weapon or Hydrogen Bomb (H Bomb) is a weapon that leverages a fusion reaction.

Dirty Bombs/ radiological weapons: bombs made of non-nuclear materials which are employed to disperse radioactive materials

The Atomic Bomb

The designs for nuclear weapons are classified into two main varieties:

Pure fission weapons

The only thing they use is uranium-238 to generate fuel. They also produce huge quantities of energy as they degrade.

Nuclear weapons are made to start an explosive chain reaction. an explosion of nuclear energy can elevate the temperature surrounding it.

The primary task that designers must complete of such super-powerful devices is the rapid assembly using fissile materials - a mixture of the uranium (or plutonium) that's been refined into "weapon-grade." Large proportions (over 50 of the population) requires only enough neutrons gathered from Chain reactions to form larger chunks inside itself when each explosion has gone off and as long as there is plenty of them available at any time the whole thing is fine since each piece is able to be used as fuel cells. This is referred to as the nuclear chain reaction.

Fission weapons that are boosted

They're a kind of nuclear weapon which makes use of the process of fusion to provide an additional source of fuel to increase dramatically the speed of splitting. The neutrons emitted through this method provide more insight into the neutrons released from conventional fissions. This allows the faster and more powerful discharge of power.

Although this is an efficient method to make an even more powerful nuclear weapon but it does come with certain risk. Fusion can be unpredictable, and if it is not controlled properly it could lead to that the weapon to go off early or not explode at all. In addition, using the fusion process as a source of fuel can make it difficult to stop the explosive that is triggered so that enhanced fission weapons are generally more safe and are more unstable in comparison to conventional fission bombs.

The Thermonuclear Weapon or Hydrogen Bomb

The Thermonuclear Weapon also known as Hydrogen Bomb is the most effective weapon that has ever been invented. It's a lot greater than the nuclear bomb, and is capable of destroying the entire city in just one explosion. The thermonuclear weapon first invented through those in United States during the Cold War to ward off from the Soviet Union from attacking America and its allies. The weapons of today remain in the hands of both Russia and the United States and Russia and constitute a significant part of their arsenals nuclear.

The thermonuclear weapon derives its name due to the fact that it utilizes thermal fusion or thermonuclear reactions in order to generate its enormous explosion force. Through a thermonuclear reaction two hydrogen atoms are combined to create one atom of Helium. The result is a huge release of energy, in the form heat. This heat will cause that thermonuclear weapon to explode.

In the simplest terms, a thermonuclear weapon functions in the following manner:

1.) A tiny fission explosive is detonated (primary step).

2.) The blast produced by the initial stage supplies the power to compress the fusion fuel which is then subjected to an atomic fission process. In the end, it reaches the temperatures required to start an atomic nuclear reaction (secondary stage).

3.) The energy generated from the secondary stage is burning the fuel and creates an fusion reaction chain.

4.) The second stage of the bomb could be protected by an additional source of fuel that could detonate, triggering an explosive reaction by neutrons generated from second stage.

First thermonuclear weapons to be tested through authorities in the United States in 1952. The weapon, known as"Mike," was the name given to it by its creators "Mike" bomb produced an output of 10.4 megatons. It was 1000 times stronger than atomic bombs dropped by Hiroshima or Nagasaki. It was Mike bomb was so massive that it was released from a balloon, instead of an aircraft.

In the years since development of thermonuclear weapons has seen many advancements in the field of fusion. The advancements have resulted in less bulky and smaller weapons that are delivered through airplanes, missiles or even aircrafts.

Dirty Bombs/radiological weapons

A dirty bomb, also known as a radiological dispersal device is untested weapon of radiological technology that blends the explosive properties of radioactive materials with those used in conventional explosions. The idea is to spread radioactive matter over an extensive region by using the traditional component, which results in contamination of the region.

There's no consensus about the efficacy of dirty bombs. Certain experts think that a blast could result in only minor physical harm, however the radioactive contamination may pose a health risk for the long term and trigger panic in the general population. Others believe that dirty bombs are more potent in their use as psychological weapons rather than actually weapon with mass destruction.

The risk of dirty bombs was recently raised from terrorist groups like Al Qaeda. The year 2001 was the time when al Qaeda operative Abu Zubaydah was arrested and questioned about plans for a nuclear attack. In 2003 the US government released a statement warning al Qaeda might be planning to employ a bomb that was dirty in the event of an attack.

Despite concerns over explosives that are dirty, there has ever been an attack that has succeeded with one.

They are usually regarded as weapons of mass disruption, rather that explosives of mass destruction because their main goal isn't killing individuals, but rather to create massive panic and damage to the economy. However, based on the level of sophistication and effectiveness of the device as well as the quantity and kind of radioactivity that is released, the use of a dirty bomb may result in serious health issues or even death.

In which nuclear weapons are kept

It is believed that the United States is believed to store its nuclear weapons stocks within a variety of underground bunkers as well as storage facilities spread across the country. The precise location of these locations are kept secret yet it is understood that they are scattered across military bases and various other safe locations.

The U.S. government has never publicly acknowledged the existence of the nuclear weapons storage facilities However, they've been widely reported in journalists and confirmed by former officials in the administration. The assumption is that the majority of America's nuclear arsenal are stored in secure locations.

The goal of these places is to keep nuclear weapons safe and secured and guarantee that they will be immediately accessed in the case in the event of an emergency situation. These locations remain secret, and only known to select high-ranking federal officials.

The presence of nuke storage facilities is a sign of the graveness of the risk to nuclear warfare. The reality that the United States has such a vast arsenal of nuclear weapons as well as the fact their distribution throughout the nation makes obvious that the federal government is contemplating the possibility of nuclear war extremely seriously.

The exact location of United States' nuclear weapon storage facilities remain private, it's important to keep in mind that the weapons are being stored to safeguard the American nation and its security interests. They should not be utilized except for the situations that are most dangerous, and it is our hope that they will never be utilized.

Additionally, Russia stores nuclear bombs within its borders. Most of them are located located in Siberia. The amount of nuclear weaponry Russia has is not known because it is a secret state matter. But, according to varying estimations, Russia has about 7 000 nuclear warheads. The US have around 6500.

Both countries have been working to reduce their arsenals of nuclear weapons after the end in the Cold War in 1991. In the year 2010, US President Barack Obama along with his Russian counterpart Dmitry Medvedev signed the New START agreement that obligated both sides to decrease the amount of nuclear arsenals they have.

The New START agreement limits each country to 800 strategic warheads that are deployed and 700 bombers and missiles deployed. The agreement also limits on the quantity of launchers every country is allowed to have at 700. This agreement took effect in

February of 2011 and is expected to run for 10 years.

Although both the United States and Russia have taken steps to lessen their nuclear arsenals, many nations around the globe are increasing their stockpiles. China, India, and Pakistan are thought to have substantially increased their arsenals of nuclear weapons in the past few years.

The increasing use of nuclear weaponry is a major global issue that has to be dealt with. In addition, the fact that many countries have nuclear arsenals makes the threat of a nuclear conflict much greater as it was in those times of Cold War.

It is crucial for all nations to collaborate to stop the spread of nuclear weapons as well as to decrease the stockpiles of deadly weapons.

Chapter 2: The Dangers Of Nuclear Weapons

Nuclear weapons are among the most hazardous weapons used in the world. They could cause huge destruction, and their impact could last for a long time. They are also costly to manufacture and use lots of resources. Small nuclear bombs may cause significant damages, while bigger ones are more likely to cause damage.

Nuclear bombs pose a risk as they release large amounts of energy once they explode. It is released through radiation, light and heat radiation. The energy generated by a nuclear explosion is so powerful that it could ignite fires and the light may be so bright, it could result in blindness. Radiation of a nuclear blast could cause cancer as well as different health problems.

Nuclear bombs can also be hazardous due to the explosions they produce. It is caused when the nuclear weapon releases radioactive particles to the air. The particles are then breath in by humans and could cause health problems. Also, fallout could contaminate drinking water as well as food items, and can make it unfit to eat or drink.

It is crucial to keep in mind that nuclear weapons are extremely hazardous weapons that are only used in the last instance. It is only appropriate to use them only when there is no alternative option to accomplish the objective. Nuclear weapons should not be handled lightly and the use of them should be considered with care.

Even tiny nuclear bombs could result in a great deal of destruction. It was the case when United States dropped two nuclear bombs over Japan in World War II. The bombs claimed the lives of thousands of Japanese and destroyed whole cities. The consequences of these bombs remain in the air today since many who were exposed to radiation of the bombs are suffering from cancer as well as various health issues.

The larger nuclear bombs are more deadly. It is estimated that there are 15,000 nuclear warheads on the world. And each one is stronger than those that were used during World War II. If even a small fraction of these were employed, it could be an all-encompassing disaster. A nuclear war could cause massive destruction, which could lead to the death of millions.

Nuclear weapons are extremely dangerous that they must not be employed. The possibility of them creating an international catastrophe is too much. States with nuclear weapons have to take every step they can to ensure they are safe and ensure they're not utilized.

Do nuclear bombs have the ability to be snatched up?

Nuclear missiles are engineered to be extremely effective in creating damage. As they are, intercepting the missiles is a challenge. There are numerous reasons that can make intercepting difficult such as the rate at which nuclear weapons move, their tiny dimensions, as well as the fact that they could be assisted with decoys and other security measures.

Missile defense systems were created to solve this problem However, they're not 100% foolproof. There have been instances like in the Gulf War, missiles were successfully stopped. There is however no guarantee that each nuclear missile will be stopped.

The best method to safeguard against nuclear weapons is by deterrence. That means a robust sufficient capability to retaliate if prospective adversaries think the risks for launching an attack are greater than the rewards. The nuclear-armed nations have worked to keep this equilibrium for several decades and has generally been effective in preventing the possibility of nuclear conflict.

Despite the risks that nuclear weapons pose, it's crucial to consider that they've only ever been employed twice in the history of mankind and both were to put an ending to wars. The future is uncertain, but it could be that nuclear weapons will be utilized in a targeted manner to meet specific goals but without creating massive destruction. But, for as the nuclear arsenal continues to exist in the world, there's always the possibility of using them to cause devastating harm.

Can nuclear bombs cause tsunami

Nuclear weapons are among the most destructive and deadly weapons ever invented. They are able to destroy entire cities and millions of people at a time. Can they cause the tsunami?

Yes, the nuclear explosion can create tsunamis. Actually, this was demonstrated for the first time during the United States' testing of nuclear weapons in the Pacific Ocean during the 1950s. The tests proved that nuclear explosions were able to cause massive waves, often hundreds of feet tall.

It should however be noted that not every nuclear explosions are likely to cause tsunamis. The power and size of the explosion are key elements, along with the depth of the water at which the explosion takes place. Furthermore, landmasses that are close to the explosion can influence whether or not the tsunami will be created.

However however, there is no doubt that nuclear bombs possess the capability of causing tsunami. Another reason that these weapons pose a risk and shouldn't be utilized.

Can nuclear bombs be?

Atomic bombs are among the most deadly weapons around the world. They could cause massive destruction and destruction, making an extremely dangerous danger to the security of the world. What is the maximum distance the bombs go?

The answer is contingent on several factors that include the kind of the bomb as well as its way of delivery. For example intercontinental ballistic missiles (ICBMs) may carry nuclear warheads across vast distances, and may be able to reach any target anywhere on the planet. Similar to cruise missiles, cruise missiles could also have nuclear warheads. They can also are capable of spanning several thousands of kilometers.

Different delivery techniques like aircrafts or ships, also have the capability of transporting nuclear bombs for large distances. There is no limit to the distance a nuclear weapon can travel as long as it's delivered using an appropriate delivery method.

But, the power of a nuclear device is not the only element that decides its destructive capability. the yield (or explosive force) of the bomb is another important aspect to consider. The atomic bomb dropped by Hiroshima was able to yield about 15 kilotons (15,000 tonnes) and the latest US nuclear tests involved bombs that yielded as high as 1 megaton (1 million tonnes).

The power to destroy nuclear weapons also depend on the location of the target. If the area of target is an urban zone, the consequences will be more destructive than if the targeted area is a rural one or an open area. The reason for this is that structures and buildings can increase the destruction of the explosion which can cause more damage as well as the loss of lives.

Nuclear weapons have become a huge worldwide concern due to the power of destruction they unleash. It is crucial to keep in mind that the power and effectiveness of these weapons are just one aspect of the equation. The kind of target as well as the way of delivering are important factors in determining the dangers a nuclear weapon is.

Who is the strongest nuclear bomb on the planet?

The most powerful nuclear bomb on the planet is B83 that was created in the United States. The B83 thermonuclear weapon is capable of the highest output in the range of 1.2 megatons (Mt) which is, 1.2 million tonnes of TNT. The B83 is considered to be a "strategic" bomb which means that it's specifically designed for use against targets that are large and hardened like military bases and chemical factories.

The second strongest nuclear bomb on the planet is the Russian "Tsar Bomba" (also called"the "King of Bombs"). The hydrogen bomb can produce an output of 50 million tonnes which translates to 50 million tons of TNT. Tsar Bomba Tsar Bomba was tested in 1961. It is considered to be the most powerful nuclear weapon that has ever used to be detonated.

The third-highest rated nuclear weapon is the B61-12. It is a bomb designed for tactical use from the United States. The weapon can have a production in the range of 0.3-0.4 Mt (300-400 kilograms). It is intended to defend against smaller and more vulnerable targets, including enemy tanks or infantry.

These are currently the three strongest nuclear bombs that exist. But, it must be emphasized that there exist several other nuclear weapons having yields much lower than those three weapons. As an example that the W76 warhead - transported in U.S. Trident II missiles is a weapon with the yield of 100 kilotons (0.1 million tonnes). The result is still a huge explosion, but the size is smaller than that of the B83 and Tsar Bomba.

Chapter 3: Humans Are Impacted By Nuclear Bombs

Nuclear weapons are among the most deadly weapons available on the planet. The consequences of a nuclear weapon on human beings can be catastrophic. Exposed to blasts or radiation, as well as the heat could cause severe injury or even death.

The results of nuclear weapons are influenced by a variety of variables, such as the dimensions of the bomb and the fission type reaction (uranium or plutonium) and the height that it detonates as well as the conditions of the weather at the time.

If a nuclear weapon is released, a huge explosion happens. The blast waves from the explosion may cause severe destruction to buildings as well as other buildings. The heat generated by the explosion may also trigger fires that could quickly spread and cause destruction to huge regions.

The radiation released by a nuclear weapon can be very harmful to humans. Exposed to high levels of radiation could cause illness and the death of a person. Radioactive isotopes, in fact, are released into the air and may travel a long distance from the site of the explosion. The isotopes could contaminate the water and food sources Exposure to them could cause severe illness or even death. Long-term effects from radiation exposure aren't completely researched, but it's believed that radiation exposure can cause an increase in the risk of getting cancer as well as other illnesses.

Anyone who is close to the explosion site at the time an explosive nuclear weapon explodes, is at chance of being injured or dying. People who are further away from the site of blast could still be at risk of ailments or injuries resulting from the fallout or radiation from the blast.

There's no safe distance to stay away from the nuclear explosion. One way to safeguard yourself from the dangers of a nuclear weapon is to seek refuge immediately following the blast.

Nuclear bombs can be extremely hazardous weapon, and the impact of nuclear weapons to humans could be devastating. It is crucial to know the threats these weapons can pose and take the necessary measures to safeguard you and your family members should there be the threat of nuclear war.

The effects of nuclear radiation are internally and externally radiated.

External contamination occurs when individuals have exposure to a high level of radiation that originates that are not within their body, like an nuclear power plant, or from a nuclear explosion.

Internal contamination happens in the event that radioactive material enters the body via the air, water or contact with the skin and accumulate in tissues. The risk is higher if individuals close to nuclear explosives or when they consume unclean food or drink polluted water.

The two types of exposure to radiation may cause serious health effects which include cancer as well as the death. It's the reason it's so important to know the hazards and steps you can take to shield you and your loved ones from radiation.

Apart from the previously mentioned kinds of contamination, it's important to mention the third type of contamination. It is known as radiation exposure that occurs when radioactive substance creates waves or particles that enter the human body. The exposure to radiation does not necessarily imply contamination, since it is only possible if the radioactive substance is in contact with the human body (externally or internal).

Similar to external and internal contaminants radioactive exposure could cause grave health issues.

Nuclear bombs: possible targets

As tensions increase between nuclear power nations around the globe and their nuclear adversaries, it is crucial to be aware of the targets that could be hit by an attack with nuclear weapons. While nobody can tell the exact location the exact location where nuclear weapons could fall, there's a few areas which are more likely to be hit over other locations.

The most probable potential targets for a nuclear attack include major cities. The reason for this is that cities are highly populated which means that a nuclear attack will cause widespread destruction and possibly death. In addition, the major cities are frequently home to prominent politicians and leaders in the military which makes them desirable targets for a hostile force.

A different target for any nuclear attack is the army base of the enemy. This could mean the missile silos of air bases as well as naval structures. A strike on these targets will limit an adversary's capabilities to wage war, and may also cause significant collateral damages.

Additionally, nuclear bombs can be employed to attack an opponent's infrastructure. These could be power stations as well as water treatment facilities as well as transportation systems. In the event of destruction, these targets could have devastating effects on the ability of a nation to function, and may cause chaos and discord.

The potential targets of nukes are numerous but it's essential to consider that every location is susceptible. It's essential to prepare to be ready for any eventuality, and try to believe in the best.

Although there's no method to be certain the exact location where nuclear weapons could be dropped from, knowing possible targets is crucial. If you know the places where the most likely targets are for being targeted the public will be more equipped in the event in the event of any attack.

The bomb was not exploded until before the attack.

In the event that a nuclear bomb gets ignited, the explosion could cause catastrophic damages to the infrastructure as well as people throughout the world. To reduce the damage caused by such an catastrophe, it's important to prepare for the worst and adopt the necessary steps.

The first step is to create a refuge in a the area where you are able to protect yourself from radiation and radiation.

In addition, it is essential to supply safe water. Contaminated water is a prime source of spreading diseases.

The third is that you'll need food items that last many days or even weeks because emergency services can become overwhelmed following the effects of an incident.

Fourthly, good hygiene is vital to preventing transmission of disease, therefore be sure to keep lots of soap and fresh garments.

In addition, having a reliable power source is essential in case you have to depend on batteries or generators to power an electrical blackout. With these easy steps, you will be able in ensuring your security as well as your wellbeing in the case that a nuclear bomb explodes.

Let's discuss each of the topics mentioned.

Shelter

There are a variety of alternatives that are available for the most appropriate method to protect yourself from nuclear blast.

Sheltering in Place

It is essential to have a place to shelter so that it is safe from radiation and the blast.

One of the most crucial aspects to consider when selecting a shelter is its capacity to guard you against harmful effects from blasts as well as radiation.

To this end it is important to consider the following outcomes from a nuclear blast:

Blast: The explosion boosts atmospheric pressure.

The force of the wind is created due to the growth of the gas spread through the blast.

Radiation: pulses of RF and gamma rays generated through the explosion

The heat generated by the fireball

Radioactive particles, fallout generated in the aftermath of nuclear blasts

Core debris are radioactive fragments of bomb fuel which have not ignited and are extremely radioactive

There are two primary kinds of shelters: above ground shelters and shelters below ground.

Above ground shelters are typically constructed of brick or concrete they are built to safeguard your from radiation and blast damage. radiation and blasts.

Shelters below ground are typically constructed of concrete or metal and can be more effective at safeguarding against radiation.

In the event that shelters are required to provide security from all of negative effects that can result from the nuclear explosion The best choice is a below-ground shelter since it is protected from all of the consequences.

Additionally, it's crucial to select a place with enough space to be able to house all of the members that are part of your family.

It is also important to think about the location of your shelter since it must be near your residence.

When you've decided to build the shelter you want to use, it's essential to fill the place with water, food as well as other necessities that should be sufficient for a minimum of two weeks.

Also, you should be prepared for the way you'll reach the shelter.

Mass care shelter

A mass care shelter can be described as temporary shelter which provides vital services for disaster victims. Mass care shelters are either private or public and are usually run by government departments, non-profit organisations, or religious organizations. Shelters for mass care provide shelter in a safe and clean place that disaster victims can stay within while waiting for an arrangement for permanent housing to be put in place. The services offered by mass care shelters are food, showers laundry facilities, medical treatment.

The sheltering of mass care can mean sharing a space with a lot of people the same space. This could be a challenge and even unpleasant.

Make sure you have the necessary cleaning supplies including soap, toothbrush, toothpaste and an outfit change. The survivors of disasters should be aware of their personal hygiene requirements during their stay at a massive health shelter.

There are many shelters that allow service animals to stay, however there are shelters for public use and even hotels that do not allow pets to stay inside. Find the safe area to bring your pets prior to disasters or emergencies occur.

Stay-at-Home

If you're unable to the luxury of an underground bunker, you should try to locate a solid structure which has thick walls to protect you from blast waves. When you've located a suitable shelter, you must cover all doors and windows with duct tape and plastic sheeting for a airtight seal.

It is also possible to remain at home, since staying inside is an option when there's no other option to protect yourself from the threat of nuclear explosion.

Water

One of the most crucial actions you can take to be prepared for a nuclear explosion is to ensure you have plenty of fresh, clean water. Most preppers suggest storing more than one gallon of drinking water per day for every person. Consider storing at least three gallons a each day to ensure hygiene and cookware.

It may appear to be a huge task to hold the water in all of that but it can be an important difference in the outcome of life or death in a situation of situation of emergency.

It is crucial to note that these guidelines are applicable to all scenarios prior to the impact of nuclear radiation.

Even during an emergency nuclear it is bottled water that will be the only option that's uncontaminated.

For those who are interested Here's how you can discover, gather, cleanse and then store the water in a way that you're ready.

Find Water

When you're camping in the wild or staying in your home, having access safe water is crucial to safety. Here are a few tips on how to locate water that you can count on during an emergency

One of the easiest methods to locate water is by searching at natural sources such as rivers, lakes and lakes. If you're in the wild they can prove to be lifesavers. It's crucial to keep in mind that all water you come across in the wilderness will have to be treated prior before you consume it. Boiling is the ideal method to get rid of bacteria and make the water safe for drinking.

Another possibility is to gather rainwater. This is done using a tarp, or any other impermeable fabric to capture rain. When you've collected the rainwater, it needs to be cleaned before drinking it. The easiest way to accomplish this is to use the coffee filter.

If you're sitting inside your house in case of situation of emergency, the best way to prepare is to store up bottles of water prior to time. This ensures that there is enough water that is clean for the duration of the emergency until it has been resolved.

The most crucial factors to be considered when gathering water is the quality of the water source. If you're making use of a groundwater source ensure that you check for contamination prior to using it. Sources of surface water including lakes and rivers should be likewise tested prior to use. After you've determined the source of water is safe then you are able to start collecting water.

In the event of an crisis, every drop water is important. This is why it's crucial to have some water collection devices for the occasion that tap water shut off or is damaged. Water collection systems come in a variety of shapes and sizes, ranging from small containers for emergencies to larger barrels. They are made from metal, plastic, as well as glass. Whatever material you decide to use, make certain that the water purifier is food-grade and free of BPA. This ensures that the water it holds can be safe to consume. If you reside in an area that's susceptible to natural catastrophes, it's an excellent idea to put the water tank inside your garage or basement. So, you'll be able to get access to safe drinking water even in the event that your electricity goes out.

There are several options that could be employed to gather water. This includes buckets, hand pumps and troughs. Each one has its benefits and drawbacks, therefore it's important to pick the best one that meets the needs of your situation. Hand pumps are generally utilized for water collection on a small scale however buckets and troughs can be used for bigger amounts of water.

When you've obtained your water and bottled it, you must put it away in a safe, safe container. Make sure you label the containers to are aware of the water that you can consider safe to drink, and which can be used for other reasons, like cooking or washing. The water that's been processed with chemicals like chlorine is required to be labeled in a clear manner and kept away in a separate container from any other source of drinking water.

By following these guidelines with these tips, you'll be able to ensure that you'll be able to access clean water even in an emergency.

Chapter 4: Get Water From Municipal Sources

Although it's true there are numerous ways to gather and purify water from the outdoors however, the methods are slow and insecure. The best option is to tap into the municipal water supply. With some planning you are able to easily connect to these water sources for drinking water that is potable, when there is an outage in power. One of the best ways to prepare is to fill large containers with water prior to when the crisis arrives. In this way, you'll always have fresh water available and not have to think about the purification. A different option is to buy an encapsulated gravity-fed water filtering system. They rely on gravity to move water through a set of filters. They will provide water that is clean and potable water. Furthermore, a lot of water supply systems in the municipal system now include fluoride which helps in preventing tooth decay. When you make use of these sources it is possible to ensure that your family and you can always access safe drinking water.

Everyday, we rely on the municipal water supply for cooking, drinking as well as cleaning. We are confident that the public institutions responsible for monitoring that our water is of high quality is working hard to shield us from harmful toxic substances. Sometimes, however, harmful toxins get through the cracks and get into our drinking water. If this occurs you must be aware of the steps you can take to safeguard yourself as well as your loved ones. To begin, determine the extent to which your water supply been affected. The information you need is available at your local government office or water company. If you have a concern you should avoid tap water for cooking, drinking and cleaning your teeth. Use bottled water, or water that's been simmered for a minimum of three minutes. It is also important to clean the surfaces you have come into contact with the contaminated water. Cleansing and disinfecting them regularly surfaces will prevent spreading of toxic substances. With these measures it will protect you as well as your family members from harm.

What do you need to know when municipal water has been contaminated?

The most crucial actions you can take to ensure yourself from illness is to make sure that your water is safe. Water contamination is an issue that affects many people, and municipal water sources are susceptible to contamination by dangerous microbes or chemical. If you think the water you use isn't safe to drink, there are couple of steps you could take to safeguard yourself. The first step is to figure whether there are any recent instances of contaminants in the water supply of your neighborhood. It is also possible to get your water tested for contamination at your local laboratory. If you do not want to drink the water you could purify it with an in-home filter system or boil it at least for three minutes. With these basic precautions will help ensure that you and your family are safe from dangers posed by contamination of drinking water.

Techniques to purify water

Anyone who is a survivalist recognizes that water is one of the most essential things to carry when you are in a situation of survival. You need water to keep hydrated, it can also be employed to cook, wash as well as for other purposes. In reality, situations of survival often occur in areas where water source isn't safe to consume. When this happens it's crucial that you know how to clean the water so that it is safe.

One of the main aspects to be aware of when dealing with emergencies is the fact that water has to be cleansed before it can be utilized.

1.) Boiling water

One of the most commonly used ways to purify water is to boil the water. It eliminates harmful viruses and bacteria and makes drinking water safe for drinking. But, it's important to simmer the water for at least one minute (for heights between 6500 and 6000 feet) or for 3 minutes (for higher altitudes) in order to make sure all contaminants have been eliminated.

Most people think boiling the water in a pot is the most effective option to clean it up However, this isn't all the time. Although boiling water kills the majority of viruses and bacteria but it is not able to eliminate every contaminant. As an example boiling water can't take out heavy metals, for example arsenic and lead and harmful chemical substances, for example, chlorine. Furthermore boiling water may increase the concentration of contaminants for instance, fluoride. Therefore, it is crucial to understand the disadvantages of boiling water prior to using it for purification purposes.

Boiling is a straightforward and effective method of purifying water. When you bring water to a simmering boil for just one minute, you will eliminate the majority of viruses and bacteria. Boiling can be particularly effective in regions where the quality of water is in question, for example those with poor sanitation infrastructure. Boiling is also an excellent option in emergency situations where there is no clean water available. Although boiling can be a powerful way to purify water however, there are some negatives. The water that is boiled tends to be bland. an unpleasant taste and can remove several minerals naturally found in the water. This is why many individuals opt to clean their water by using different methods like filtration, or ultraviolet light. These methods do make no difference to the taste or composition the water.

Important: Boiling water from the tap is not a good way to eliminate radioactive matter during nuclear emergency. Make sure you have water that has been boiled as well as bottles of water on hand in case of emergency in case of nuclear disaster.

2) Bleach

To cleanse water by bleach, just include eight drops of bleach for every gallon. The solution is well stirred and then let it rest for 30 mins before using. This is a great method in situations of emergency when there isn't access to pure water. Be aware that bleach could be hazardous in the event of ingesting it, so make certain to keep the product away from animals and children. If used correctly it is an easy and effective method to cleanse water.

A lot of people believe bleach to be a reliable means of purifying water. It is however efficient at killing bacteria but not viruses. To perform its job, it needs to be utilized in large amounts and the contact time is required to be extended and isn't suitable to purify large amounts of water. Furthermore, bleach could affect the health of humans when consumed in large quantities. In light of this, it is essential to employ alternative methods to purify water such as boiling water or filtering.

Water filtering methods

There's an array of ways to cleanse water, however they each work the same manner. Water passes through a filtering medium like sand or charcoal that traps impurities as well as harmful substances. This method can eliminate many of the harmful substances found in water. These include the viruses, bacteria and protozoa. The process is typically utilized in conjunction with other methods for purification including chlorination in order to guarantee that the water you drink is safe to consume. Even though it's not completely absolute, it is an effective method to eliminate the majority of contaminants in the water.

The most popular sort of water filter is the activated carbon filtration system made to eliminate impurities like chemical and chlorine from the water you drink. Another option to consider is reverse osmosis water filter. It utilizes a semi-permeable membrane that helps get rid of dissolved solids as well as contaminants from your water. Additionally ultraviolet light filters can be efficient in killing virus and bacteria, making an ideal option in households with young animals or children. There are so many choices to select from, understanding the various types of water filters will help you choose the best filter for your home.

1.) Gravity filters

There are a variety of different kinds of water filtration systems available on the market. Water filters that are gravity-based is one type of filter that makes use of gravity to pull water through several filtering stages. One of the advantages of gravity water filtering is the fact that they are able to be operated without power and are a good solution in times of emergency or in locations where power is not available. The typical gravity filter consists of an upper chamber in which the dirty water is stored and a lower one where water filtered by the filter is stored. The water flows through the filter via gravity. When it goes through various filters, the impurities are eliminated and pure water is collected within the bottom chamber. Gravity filtering can differ in terms of size and complexity but they all have a common purpose of supplying clean and safe drinking water.

2.) Filters for water vs purifiers

In terms of the emergency preparedness of your home water is among the most essential things to keep on hand. However, what is the best method to make sure you've got safe, clean water available in any emergency? Filters and purifiers for water provide both efficient ways to purify water, however they operate differently.

Water filters eliminate impurities in water through the physical trapping of them within a filtration. It can also be used to get rid of bacteria, sediment as well as other harmful substances. Water purifiers in contrast make use of chemical or ultraviolet radiation to eliminate the contaminants. They are therefore powerful against viruses, which aren't large enough to be absorbed by filters.

What is the better option? The answer is dependent on what you need. If you're planning for an emergency it is important to understand what kinds of contaminants you're likely to come across. If you're looking for security in general and peace of mind, water filters are an excellent option. However, if you're seeking the most comprehensive level of protection, then a purifier is the best way to choose.

Chapter 5: Alternative Methods To Purify Water

1) Iodine

Iodine is a chemical element that has the symbol I and the atomic code 53. It's a yellowish solid non-metal with an luster of metallic. Purely, it's Odorless however, when used in commercial applications it does have a mild scent like bleach. Iodine can be used in a variety of diverse ways, the most popular of that is to cleanse water. This is done by adding a couple of drops of iodine in the water, and then waiting for it to rest for about 30 minutes before drinking. Iodine can kill organisms or viruses that may be that are present in the water which makes it safe to consume. In addition, it can be used to clean the water to be stored by mixing it into the water after which seal the container. This ensures that the water is pure as well as safe to drink over longer periods of time.

2.) Carbon filtering activated

There are numerous methods of filtration water. One that is the most efficient is made by the use of activated carbon. Activated Carbon filters are commonly utilized by survivalists and preppers since they provide the most reliable method of get rid of impurities in water. The process of activated Carbon filtering is quite simple. water passes through an activated carbon that is able to absorb impurities like chlorine, chemicals as well as heavy metals. This means that the filtering water is pure and safe to consume. Apart from functioning as an efficient water purifier, activated carbon can also serve many other benefits. It's a great way to cleanse air, eliminate toxic substances from your body as well as treat specific ailments. It is the most important tool for those who is interested in self-reliance or preparedness.

3) Reverse Osmosis

Recently there's an increasing desire to prepare for catastrophe scenario. One of the biggest actions that preparedness professionals can take is stockpile water. However, in an environment where the water supply is becoming increasingly polluted What can you do to be confident that the stored water is safe to consume? A solution is to cleanse the water you drink by using an reverse osmosis filter. Reverse osmosis filtering works by pushing the water into a semipermeable membrane and leaving the pollutants in the water. In the end, they can remove the impurities like virus, bacteria and heavy metals out of the water you drink. Furthermore reverse osmosis systems can remove solids that are dissolved like salt that could make the water you store tasting better. In case you're planning for disaster, or simply seeking to improve the taste of the water you drink reverse osmosis filters can be an ideal option.

4) ION Exchange

Ion exchange is the process which involves the exchange of ions between two materials to cleanse water. A typical method of preparing is to fill water jugs and keep for the eventuality in the event of power interruptions. ION exchange refers to a form of water treatment process that helps eliminate harmful substances from water. It works by transferring the ions in the affected water for the ions from the treated solution. The most popular form that uses ION exchange happens with sodium that is a method of exchange for sodium ions that are present in the water for ions of chloride. It is efficient in eliminating a variety of pollutants, such as radionuclides, heavy metals organic compounds, and radionuclides. ION exchange is an extremely popular method of water treatment because it's highly efficient and customizable to get rid of specific contaminants. A ION exchange system will aid in removing the impurities in water and make it safe to drink during situations of emergency. Furthermore they have a low maintenance requirement and need minimal maintenance. This makes they a fantastic choice for both non-preppers and preppers alike.

Techniques to test water

There are many ways to test the water's quality. The kind of water to be test (e.g. drinking water, wastewater or even surface water) as well as the information desired will help determine which technique to employ. Most commonly, methods used include the use of microscopes, chemical analysis as well as biological tests. Chemical analysis is the process of looking for certain substances like heavy metals, or pesticides. A microscope examination may reveal that there are bacteria and other microorganisms. Biochemical tests employ indicators to determine the level of pollution which can harm people's health. Every method comes with its strengths and weaknesses, and it's important to pick the best method to deal with the particular situation.

If you are in a situation of crisis, the best method to assess the water's quality is using home tests kits.

If you're concerned about the health of the water you drink If you are concerned about the quality of your drinking water, consider purchasing the water test kit at an appliance or home improvement retailer. Although the exact instructions will be different depending on the manufacturer but the overall procedure is fairly straightforward. Start by obtaining a sample of clean water into a container. After that put the reagent you purchased comes in the kit. Add it to the water. Stir it to mix thoroughly. Then, you can compare the hue of the water to the graph available to establish the amount of contaminants in. Though tests for water quality aren't completely reliable, they do offer a basic impression of whether or not your drink is safe.

There are many water quality tests that are accessible to customers. One of the most commonly used types of test to determine water quality is a test for bacteria. The test is designed to determine the contamination of harmful microorganisms within water.

Another kind of test for water quality is the chemical test. The test is designed to determine the presence of toxic chemicals present in the water. The third kind of test for water quality is physical tests. The test is designed to determine the presence of physical pollutants in water. Each kind of test for water quality at home offers its own advantages as well as drawbacks. The tests for bacteria are typically the most reliable, however they can cost a lot. Chemical tests are cheaper however, they're less accurate than test for bacteria. Physical tests are among the most expensive but are also the most inaccurate.

If the results from the test is positive It means that there aren't any hazardous contaminants that are present within the drinking water. This is great news for anyone drinking the water that comes from this source. But, if the outcome is positive, this implies that there are harmful substances inside the water. It is an extremely bad news story to anyone drinking the water that comes from this source. One of the best options when the results are positive is to locate a different source for drinking water. There are a variety of ways to achieve this, including the use of a water purifier or purifier, or boiling the water prior to drinking it. No matter what method you pick ensure that you and your family members are safe from danger by drinking clean water and safe water.

The first 30 minutes: Close your eyes, and cover your face

The first light produced by the nuclear explosion could cause brief blindness as well as burning injuries that are severe. You should stay as as far away from the site of the explosion as you can. If you aren't able to, safeguard your eyes by keeping them clear and securing your face by putting your arm around.

For instance the A-1 megaton bomb that was dropped on Hiroshima can blind those as far as 13 miles in the event of the day that is clear and could be up to 53 miles from the site on an evening with clear skies.

First 45 minutes: Seek shelter

Stay out of the path of the blast wave If you have the basement or any other underground area, go there right away and wait until officials confirm that it's safe to go out.

If you are unable to locate underground, or you're trapped in the debris, wrap your body with as much as is possible, a sturdy doors or table such as a door, and then wait for rescuers.

The first 24 hours: Stay within

The resulting radiation of an explosion of nuclear energy is extremely risky. It could cause burned skin, radiation-related sickness or even death.

After you've entered the safe zone, you can remove the clothes that are contaminated after exposure to radiation particles. Take a shower to wash off the fallout on the skin.

Don't forget: those who were on the ground during an explosion are advised to wash whenever they can. Make sure the water is not too hot and that soap is applied with care.

Chapter 6: Treatment And Prevention Of Radiation-Related Injury And Illnesses

Emergencies in radiation can strike suddenly and without notice. These can result from natural disasters such as nuclear power plant disasters, or terrorist attack.

The exposure to radiation could damage the health of your body. They can cause damage to the DNA and cells of your body and can cause cancer. Additionally, it can cause ailments, including acne reddening, infertility birth defects, cataracts and even cataracts.

If you've been in the vicinity of radiation you have ways to ensure your health

Remove yourself from the location where radiation incident occurred as soon as is possible.

Remove all clothing and shoes which may contain radioactive substances. Put them in a closed bag.

Wash your face gently with soap and water. This will eliminate any traces of dirt.

Don't take any food or drink before you've been informed that it's safe to consume it.

Be aware of your conditions and health is crucial following a radiation-related incident. Record any health changes like nausea, diarrhea or nausea. Always get medical help in the event that you develop one of these.

The symptoms of Acute Radiation Symptoms (ARS) can consist of nausea, vomiting headache, diarrhea and loss of hair. They can manifest from several hours or days following exposure to high doses of radiation.

It is crucial to note that ARS can occur at the time:

The dose of radiation was very high.

Internal contamination was the cause.

The whole body is made visible.

It was absorbed in just a few 30 minutes.

Synthons in ARS may be separated into three distinct phases:

1.) The prodromal or the initial stage: This may be a few hours or two or three days, and can be characterized by a variety of non-specific symptoms like malaise, anorexia, fatigue, nausea diarrhoea, vomiting, and nausea.

2.) The manifest illness phase The phase starts with the development of symptoms more specific to the illness like skin reddening, erythema (reddening) as well as Oedema (swelling) or desquamation (shedding) in addition to as mucosal damage. Haematological signs like anemia thrombocytopenia (low number of platelets) as well as the leukopenia (low white blood cells count) are also possible in this stage.

3.) Phase of recovery It begins with the time that a patient's condition begins improving and could take weeks to months. The patient may suffer long-term consequences including immunosuppression and cataracts, growth retardation and the sterility.

It can cause death If not addressed quickly and efficiently. The death rate is usually within 2 to 4 weeks of the onset symptoms, and it is usually caused by haemorrhage or an infections. Treatment for ARS involves aggressive treatment within a hospital environment. There's no particular treatment to treat radiation poisoning. However the treatment of symptoms can increase the chances for living.

If you have been in the vicinity of radiation sources, it's vital to seek medical assistance immediately. Treatments for radiation exposure can comprise countermeasures or drugs which aid your body in getting rid of radioactive material. The treatments include Potassium Iodide (KI), Prussian Blue, DTPA, and Neupogen(r) (filgrastim)

Potassium Iodine: Potassium iodide (KI) is a form of salt of the stable form of iodine. It is a supplement to oral intake to block the thyroid gland's ability to absorb radioactive iodine which could release during the event of a nuclear explosion or a terrorist attack. KI is to be used in accordance with the instructions of the local and state authorities.

Prussian Blue: Prussian blue is a medicine that bonds to radioactive elements within your digestive tract so that they can get out from your body via your stool. This treatment may be administered to adults and children who've eaten (swallowed) massive quantities of radioactive cesium or Thallium.

DTPA: DTPA (diethylenetriamine pentaacetic acid) is a medication that bonds to radioactive materials within your body, so that they can pass out in your urine. The treatment is available to adults and children who are exposed to radioactive americium, plutonium or curium.

Neupogen: Neupogen (filgrastim) is a medication that assists your body create greater numbers of white blood cells. These cells fight diseases. This therapy is utilized by those who've been exposed to high levels of radiation ionizing. The side effects of these treatments generally are not severe and disappear off on their own. Some side effects may be severe. It is important to speak to your doctor regarding the potential risks and advantages of these procedures.

The most important thing is to safeguard yourself from exposure to radiation by being well-prepared. It is important to have an emergency kit that includes supplies including water, food, as well as a first aid kit.

Also, you can safeguard yourself against radiation by staying inside and staying clear of areas which are infected with radiation. If you're outdoors be sure to stay away from any object which could be affected by radiation.

Cleanse your clothes and skin well if you come in contact with any surfaces that are contaminated.

What can you do to give food to your baby

If you're a mom who is pregnant, the best method to shield your baby in case of nuclear emergencies is to keep them inside. The breastfeeding process should not be your only alternative for feeding your child. In reality there is a chance that you could be infected internalally, so the most effective solution in such situations is stop nursing for a short period of time.

Consider these options:

Use infant formula that is ready to feed since it's the most secure alternative for breastfeeding milk. It is, in fact, an sterile liquid and doesn't require to be mixed with water.

If you don't already have formula for feeding your infant then use a clean, dry sponge or towel clean any feeding equipment that may be in contact with the baby's mouth. These include pacifiers, bottles or anything else your baby is likely to put into their mouth. Make a formula for your infant that is powdered in accordance with the directions on the label, and by boiling bottled water which is cooled at least 30 minutes. Be sure to wash all food items as mentioned in the previous paragraph. Utilize commercial infant foods in the event that you are unable to prepare your own the formula. Remember to wash the feeding equipment as mentioned in the previous paragraph.

Following the explosion

In the event of a nuclear explosion then the first thing to take is to seek refuge.

Following a nuclear accident It is essential to stay inside and get refuge. Radiation emitted by the blast can be extremely dangerous and can even cause death in the event that you're exposed for excessively long.

The length of time you'll need in the shelter will be contingent upon a variety of factors, such as the magnitude of the blast and the quantity of fallout. It is recommended that the US Centers for disease control and prevention suggests staying at the shelter for a minimum of 24 hours. The fallout will have time to settle, and let you assess the situation before leaving. If you can, locate an underground shelter or has walls that are thick because this can provide an additional shield against radiation. But, 24 hours is an extremely brief amount of time when you consider the situation where there is no sources of energy stored in the shelter ahead of time.

What time and what day are you able to go out?

If you've got plenty of food and water inside your home You may not have to leave for a long time. The recommendation is to hold off for a period of 2 weeks that will allow to allow the majority of fallouts to disappear. If you must go outdoors sooner, you should protect your skin from the sun in the most effective way possible, and be sure to stay clear of breathing in dust particles. Make sure you stay away from the potential for dust fallout. If you are able use a mask, do so to ensure that the air you breathe is clean. After showering, dress in clean clothes immediately in order to eliminate any harmful substances present within your body.

Chapter 7: A Brief Lesson In History

On the 6th of August 1945, a glorious day on the streets of Hiroshima, Japan, the world was forever changed. In 1945, the United States dropped the first Atomic bomb ever dropped over the gorgeous city that killed around 140,000 inhabitants. The next day, Nagasaki was bombed, and another 70,000 would suffer the similar fate. The destruction caused by the attacks continues to affect all over the world until this day.

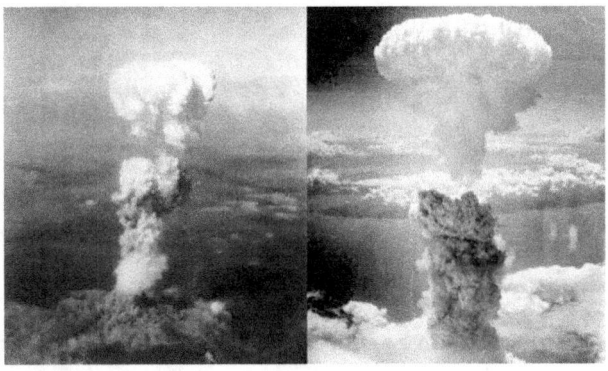

Left: Hiroshima; right: Nagasaki

The nuclear catastrophes represented a major turning point in the human story. Humanity had mastered the ability to demolish itself on an incredible size. The bombs were a brand new form of weapon, and their destruction was unimaginable.

The devastating impact of the nuclear bombs was swift and apocalyptic. The blasts immediately caused the deaths of tens of thousands and caused a massive devastation. People who survived were forced to endure the most horrific of experiences devastated houses, streets littered rubble, the stench from the dead irradiated as well as the risk from radiation illness.

The effects that lasted for a long time were damaging. A lot of survivors were affected by radiation-related sickness that led to health issues like birth defects, cancer and genetic changes. Radiation had an lasting influence on the surroundings and the residents of those affected regions.

In spite of the horrors of the attack, many believe that the bombings were needed in order to bring an end to World War II. They led to Japan's unconditional surrender and saved countless lives which would have been destroyed when an invading force invaded Japan. The morality in using nuclear weapons remains controversial and subject to controversy to this day.

The Race to Build a New Weapon

In World War II, the United States initiated the Manhattan Project that was a classified federal program designed to develop an arsenal of nuclear power ahead of Germany was able to. Physics professor Robert Oppenheimer led the project that cost more than two billion dollars and employed nearly 130,000 individuals. The success of the world's first nuclear bomb on the 16th of July 1945 at Alamogordo, New Mexico, was the beginning of the nuclear race for good.

The president Harry S. Truman ultimately made the decision to utilize the atomic bomb to bring an end to the war against Japan. The war's cost was debilitating as well, and the bomb offered the chance to swiftly stop the war. The president Truman was forced to consider the risk of loss of lives due to a long-term conflict against Japan against the devastating consequences that the use of the nuclear bomb could have. He argued that the atomic bomb was the most effective way for saving American lives.

A City Vanishes in an Instant

On the 6th of August 1945, the very first atomic bomb fell on Hiroshima. The bomb, dubbed "Little Boy," instantly killed an estimated 140,000 residents and destroyed more than 90 percent in the entire city. People who survived suffered psychological and physical marks that would last for an entire lifetime.

The next day, the 9th of August 1945, an additional atomic bomb dropped onto Nagasaki. It was dubbed the "Fat Man," caused the deaths of 70,000 and wiped out a third Nagasaki's population. The bombings achieved the intended effect and Japan was surrendered just six days after and brought an end to World War II.

Following the explosions brought a mixture of devastation, loss and destruction. The survivors were left in the aftermath of losing family members, homes and even communities. The full extent of loss was not fully realized until the end of the conflict.

A New Threat to Survivors

The radiation that was released by Atomic bombs left lasting effects on survivors. A lot of those who lived near the blast's radius experienced symptoms of radiation sickness such as nausea, vomiting, diarrhoea and loss of hair. The workers in factories close to the ground zero area were especially vulnerable to radiation sickness, and many perished in the space of a few days. But the consequences of this were numerous and far-reaching including the increase chance of developing cancer, were not completely realized for years.

The Long-Term Effects

The survivors of the bombings as well as their descendants continue to bear from the effects of their consequences nearly a century on. Apart from the immediate consequences of radiation illness, those who survived have also seen higher incidences of cancer, which includes the solid tumours and leukaemia along with other diseases like cataracts, thyroid diseases. Children born by survivors during the time following the attacks have been identified to have higher incidences of birth defects as well as developmental retardations. The effects of these have been transmitted to generations of children which serves as a stark recall of the damage caused by the nuclear bombs.

The Legacy of the Bombings

The nuclear explosions of Hiroshima and Nagasaki created a legacy which continues to resonate even to today. They marked the dawn of the age of nuclear weapons, and fear of nuclear war has posed an ongoing threat to the globe ever since. Also, the bombings sparked an arms race that was rekindled in the United States and the Soviet Union which led to the period of fear and tension known as the Cold War.

The attacks also raised significant ethical and moral questions regarding the usage of nuclear weapons during the war. The devastation caused by nuclear bombs caused many to question morality employing such destructive weapons. These bombings have also revealed the dangers associated with nuclear weapons as well as the need for international cooperation to stop any future use of nuclear weapons.

In the end, the legacy of Hiroshima along with Nagasaki is one of memorial and commemoration. This was an incredibly tragic incident that changed the face of humanity forever. Although some believe that the bombings were essential for the end of World War II, the devastating effects of the bombs is not to be missed. It is imperative to recollect the lessons that were learned from the tragedy and strive to create a world that is free nukes. In the time since the bombings, many memorials, museums, as well as ceremonies have been erected across the globe to commemorate the memories of the victims and passed away. The efforts are powerful reminders of the impact of combat and the significance in pursuing peace and also ensure that victims of the nuclear bombings won't be forgotten.

Chapter 8: Nuclear Weapons

In the center of any discussion on how to survive any nuclear attack lies the understanding of what weapons are, and the incredibly risk they pose. They are powerful weapons which make use of nuclear reactions to unleash a massive amount of energy shape of an explosive explosion. The weapons are capable to do massive harm as well as pulverize entire cities and decimate millions of individuals in just a couple of minutes.

The weaponry of nuclear war is limited to two instances in the history of mankind however, the effects of those strikes in Hiroshima as well as Nagasaki in 1945 were tragic, with lasting impacts on the health, environment and well-being of the population affected. Furthermore, in the present threats of nuclear attacks is looming in the general public, as do tensions between countries and terrorist organizations that harbor evil intentions towards the population.

In this section we'll explore the fundamentals of nuclear weapons as well as their mechanism of operation, as well as the threats they can pose. In addition, we will dispel many of the myths and misinformation about nuclear weapons, to help be aware of the dangers and plan for the most dire consequences. At the conclusion of this section, you'll be aware of the risks associated with nuclear weapons as well as the significance in being prepared for the event of a nuclear war across the globe.

What are Nuclear Weapons?

The potency of nuclear weapons is their capacity to produce an enormous amount of energy within a fraction of time. They are also known as nuclear bombs they are one of the most destructive tools that have ever been created by humans. These weapons are explosive and get their destructive power by nuclear reactions. They can happen via nuclear fission, or Fusion. Fission is a process where the nucleus in an atom breaks down into smaller pieces, which releases an enormous amount of energy. The energy is released causes an explosion. Nuclear fusion, on contrary, happens when two atomic nuclei join together and form a bigger nucleus that releases even greater energy. The power released through nuclear weapons is by magnitude more than conventional explosives. It can also cause massive damage across an extensive region.

Imagine a blast such a magnitude that it destroys all that is within its range and leaves nothing but chaos behind. That's the frightening reality of nuclear blasts.

The blast-wave that results from the nuclear explosion may devastate structures, destroy trees and create a blaze which can destroy everything that is within its path. However, it's not the only thing that happens; the explosion can also release a large amount of radiation. This is harmful for health. This can lead to extreme burns, radiation illness, or even the death of. The long-term effects from radiation exposure can cause birth defects, cancer as well as genetic changes that could be passed on over generations. The risks of an explosion of nuclear power aren't only limited to the immediate effects of the explosion. Explosions can also send massive amount of dust and other debris in the air, forming an erupting cloud of mushroom that could disperse radioactive fallout for many miles. The fallout could be harmful to water sources and food items and make it risky for the survivors to consume food and water. Another risk of nukes is radiation (EMP) generated by them. A EMP is a sudden burst of power that could destroy electronics or energy grids, leading to huge disruption and chaos. The nuclear threat is believed to trigger an atomic winter in which the blast would release lots of debris and dust to the air that it will block sunlight which would cause a rapid decrease in temperature, which could cause crop failure or hunger.

A nuclear explosion can cause a lot of trouble for anyone caught within the blast's radius.

It's crucial to know that although nuclear weapons do have the ability to cause devastating damages, there are several myths and misconceptions about their use. The most effective way to avoid in the event of a nuclear strike is to prepare and to take the necessary precautions required to guarantee survival.

Mythbusting -Myths & Facts about Nuclear Survival

Survival of nuclear war is often a subject of debate, obscured by myths and misinformation. In this section we'll break down some of the most commonly-cited misconceptions, and provide some important details about how to survive an attack from nuclear weapons.

The Top Ten Myths about Nuclear War Survival

1. Myths: "If a nuclear bomb explodes it's impossible to do to stay alive."

The fact is that with the proper methods, training and expertise You can improve the odds of being able to survive in the event of a nuclear strike.

2. The Myth "Radiation is a killer immediately."

The fact is that radiation sickness may last for weeks, or even days before it manifests, and it is possible to take measures to reduce the risk of exposure.

3. Myths: "All food and water can be affected and inedible."

A fact: Having a good stockpile as well as proven purification methods will assist you in procuring safe foods and water sources.

4. The Myth "Sheltering will not protect you from the threat of nuclear war."

The fact is that sheltering can provide the best protection against the nuclear fallout, if that you have a sufficient shelter as well as materials.

5. Mythology: "Nuclear war belongs to the history of mankind and it will never occur ever again."

The fact is that nuclear war is an unafraid possibility and it's crucial to prepare in the event of the worst scenario coming to happen.

6. Myths: "Only the wealthy can be able to afford preparing for nuclear war."

Truth: Although the existence of financial reserves can help in the development of better-quality assets, survival in nuclear conflict does not have to cost a lot of money There are plenty of economical ways of preparing for war, which we'll explore in the next chapters.

7. Myths: "You can't protect yourself from a direct nuclear explosion."

In reality, while being in the blast's radius can be fatal You can make steps to reduce their impact and enhance your chance to survive and avoid getting a meal for the blast.

8. Myths: "If society collapses after an attack on nuclear weapons then it's each man to his own."

In fact, the human nature is to function within an underlying social system. Collaboration and building community are essential for survival and reestablishing a social framework following a nuclear attack.

9. Myths: "The children and the old cannot withstand the threat of nuclear war."

The fact is that certain populations may be more susceptible to the consequences of nuclear attacks however, if they are prepared, they still stand an increased chance of surviving.

10. The Myth "Surviving the aftermath of a nuclear strike will be futile, and is unworthy of the effort."

The reality is that while the thought of nuclear war may be terrifying maintaining continuity gives an increased confidence in your control as well as boost your chances of surviving.

There are a few myths concerning nuclear safety. We'll now look at the actual factual information.

Top 10 facts about Nuclear War Survival

1. The main results of a nuclear attack include the initial blast along with thermal radiation as well as radioactive radiation.

2. Radiation from the fallout source is among the longest-lasting and most dangerous release that occurs following the nuclear explosion.

3. Shelter is vital to survive radiation from fallout.

4. Storing food, water and medical supplies is vital to survive the aftermath of a nuclear strike.

5. Exposure to radiation can cause long-term adverse health effects such as an increase in the risk of getting cancer and genetic

mutations, birth defects for newborn babies as well as other diseases.

6. Alert systems and emergency communication aid in preparing people for and respond to nuclear strike.

7. Survival in the event of nuclear war requires the combination of physical readiness along with practical experience and mental strength.

8. The survival of nuclear war isn't only an issue for individuals, it's an issue that is a collective one that demands coordination and preparation.

9. There are numerous resources to assist people in preparing in case of a nuclear strike that include the government, survivalist organizations as well as online communities for preppers.

10. Although we would like to believe that nuclear war never is a possibility, being prepared gives your peace of mind and boost

the chances of surviving any situation of emergency.

Conclusion

Survival in the event of nuclear war is an incredibly complex and difficult issue; you must learn the truths and myths concerning nuclear war survival to make educated decisions with regard to safety and security. Beware of false information and myths. Make sure you are prepared and knowledgeable, which will improve the likelihood of survival in the case of a nuclear strike.

Chapter 9: Prepare & Plan A Survival Strategy

If you want to survive an attack on nuclear weapons having a strategy is vital. If you don't have a strategy, you'll be in a panic, and take bad decisions which could put at risk your life or the life of those you love.

For a plan of action that is practical for the entire family take the following steps:

Step 1: Know the Risks and Potential Targets

As the tensions between countries increase and nations, the threat of nuke attack is becoming more apparent. We don't want to think about the repercussions of the detonation of a nuclear weapon, however to ensure that you are prepared for the worst case scenario, you must be aware of the targets that could be hit by the attack.

The identification of the targets that are likely to be hit by the possibility of a nuclear strike isn't an easy job, however it can be accomplished through thorough research and analysis. A good place to begin is to look at the military and political tensions among nations. States with a historical history of violence or conflict tend to be more likely to attack or even be targeted.

Furthermore, cities that are large as well as areas that are densely populated can be the prime targets for an attack by nuclear. Large political and financial centers and military facilities are extremely risky locations. Take note of the areas which have an important cultural or historical significance like National landmarks, or sites of worship.

However, it's not only about location, but the type of weapon employed as well as its purposeful effects could be able to provide clues to possible marks. A low yield nuclear weapon will be more likely to be utilized for a strike that is tactical, for example, against targets that are military and targets, whereas a weapon with a higher yield has a larger impact across a greater area and is likely to be utilized against an area of significant population.

How can you start to determine possible targets within your region? In the first place, be up-to-date. Be aware of current developments as well as geopolitical tensions. Be sure to follow reliable news sources as well as the government agencies which provide threats assessments as well as intelligence reports.

Consider the other infrastructural locations of your neighborhood. Do you have military facilities and power plants or public buildings in the vicinity? Are there major communications hubs, transportation hubs, or other major structures? Consider the places where people commonly congregate, for example sporting stadiums, convention centers or malls for shopping.

Also, pay attention to the surroundings. Be aware of unusual behavior or activity like strange traffic patterns, or suspicious people monitoring specific areas. Inform local law enforcement agencies or emergency management authorities.

It's not possible to determine the precise target of nuclear attacks Being aware of dangers and taking preventive measures to plan can be the difference between life or the end of your life. Be aware, be informed and remain safe.

Step 2: Decide on a Shelter Location

If a nuclear strike is likely If a nuclear attack is imminent, locating an safe place to shelter is a lifesaver. With so many information out there what can you do to be certain you're making the correct option? Stay with us, and we'll help you through choosing the right refuge to withstand the threat of nuclear war.

Know Your Surroundings

The first step towards determining the best sheltering location to become familiar with the area you are in. Consider the location of possible areas of attack, including defense installations, government buildings as well as major centres of population. This way then, you will have an understanding of the potential blast radius and fallout zones of nuclear attacks that could occur in your vicinity.

Look for Natural Shields

Nature could be your best friend when you are looking for the safe place to shelter. Find natural elements such as hills, mountains, or valleys that could provide an additional shield from radiation and blast. If possible, locate a spot which is at least a mile away from an attainable area of attack, and also provides a natural barrier between you and the target.

Seek out Professional Guidance

Get in touch with professionals in the field for more information about the most safe shelters in your region. There are several organizations that can help you. Department of Homeland Security, the Federal Emergency Management Agency (FEMA) along with local emergency management authorities will provide useful resources that can help to determine the most secure places for seeking shelter. In addition, there are a myriad of websites and applications that are available, including the FEMA app as well as the Radiation emergency medical Management app that can provide users with helpful tips and information on how to handle the aftermath of a nuclear incident.

Create a Roadmap

When you've located potential shelter sites, you need to prepare for the future. Plan how you'll arrive at the shelter, for how long it will take to stay there, as well as what equipment you'll require to store. It's suggested to store at the least two weeks worth of water, food and any other supplies you will need like first aid kits as well as equipment for monitoring radiation.

Practice Makes Perfect

The final stage in preparing for nuclear attacks is practicing your plan. Make sure you and your family are in the habit of practicing drills and make sure that everyone understands the procedure and how to reach the shelter swiftly and in a safe manner. This can help to reduce anxiety and confusion in case that there is an attack.

Step 3: Plan for Evacuation

If there is an nuclear attack Your shelter might not be sufficient to protect the family and yourself. It's essential to put an evacuation plan in order to be able to easily and without risk evacuate the area. Evacuation is a difficult job, but with a bit of pre-planning and preparation you'll be able to increase the chances of success.

Stay Informed

The very first thing to do in an evacuation plan is staying updated. It is essential to be aware of the latest details about the site and impact of the nuclear attack. Be sure to possess a battery-powered or hand-cranked radio in order to be alerted of emergencies and news. Make a list of your the emergency contact numbers and organizations in your area that include the police as well as the fire department and medical personnel.

Establish Multiple Evacuation Routes

When you've got the most up-to-date details, it is time to identify various evacuation routes. Find several ways that are out of the zone and devise different routes to get there. Take into consideration the best route to meet your family's requirements for example, avoiding congestion-ridden roads and choosing quieter back roads. Remember that some routes may be closed make alternate routes, and make sure you are prepared to modify the plans you have in place if needed.

Prepare a Go-Bag

The go-bag is an essential component of any plan for evacuation. It's a bag that's pre-packed with the essentials that you'll require to last for several days. The bag should contain essential items like a first-aid kit, non-perishable food items, additional clothing, water, blankets, flashlights, radio, batteries maps of the area, as well as cash. Store your bags in a conveniently accessible place in your home, for example near the shelter's entry point, and be sure everyone in your family knows exactly where it is.

Have a Communication Plan

Communication is vital during any evacuation. Be sure all family members are aware of how to handle if they are separated. Set up a place in the area of concern in which you are able to gather. If you can, establish one designated outside-of-town contact everyone in the family can contact to confirm their condition. It is crucial to prepare a backup plan for the event that communication systems go out of order or overloading.

Practise the Evacuation Plan

Also, practice your evacuation plan frequently. Do exercises in your home with the family members to ensure everyone is prepared in case of emergency. Modify the plan if necessary, and then update the plan according to current patterns. Practice regularly can ease stress and help ensure a successful conducted evacuation.

Conclusion

A plan for evacuation is an essential step to planning for nuclear attack. Through staying up-to-date, setting various evacuation routes, making bags for evacuation, having an evacuation plan for communication as well as practicing the routinely, you will be able to effectively move into an safe area. Be aware that in the event of an emergency situation, time is of the crucial importance. The better prepared you are in advance, the better prepared you will be to take on the challenges.

Step 4: Communication Plan

In the event of a nuclear explosion and you are a victim, it is essential to prepare a communications plan put in place to make sure that you are connected to family members and get crucial updates about the effects of the incident from authorities. Communication is vital to survive in the post-apocalyptic era and having access to accurate information could make the impact.

Devise an Emergency Communication Plan

Make a plan for emergency communications for your loved ones, family members as well as colleagues prior to it being way too for you to be late. Be sure that everyone is familiar on the strategy. Think about using different channels for communications, such as traditional paper, technology for computers as well as digital methods.

Pick a primary and backup gathering place if you become separated from your family during the incident. Choose a family or friend person who is not in the zone of attack to act as an emergency caller. The person you choose to contact can serve as the central point of contact and communicate important details to your family and other friends in the event that you are inaccessible to them.

Stay Informed

In the aftermath of a nuclear incident there will be sources of information that will be limited, and news can spread fast. You must seek out reliable facts to prevent falling to untrue claims. Make sure you have a hand-cranked or battery-powered radio that can receive notifications from emergency broadcasting devices.

If you can, visit official government websites as well as accounts on social media for up-to-date details. Keep tabs on local news channels however be cautious of untrue news reports. Keep a list of reliable sources to consult as well as your emergency contact.

Protect Your Communication Devices

Electromagnetic impulses (EMPs) generated by an explosion of nuclear energy can harm electronic gadgets, such as radios and phones. To safeguard your devices for communication put them into a Faraday cage. This is specially designed to prevent electromagnetic radiation.

It is possible to make a basic Faraday cage by covering the metal box with cardboard, and then covering your gadgets with aluminium foil. A better option is to purchase an Faraday bag. This is one that is specifically made to block electromagnetic field.

Use Caution When Communicating

In a post-apocalyptic environment it is important to be careful when you communicate. Make sure you know who you're communicating with, and stay clear of divulging sensitive information via devices like your shelter's address or any supplies.

Make use of code words or phrases in your emergency contacts for communicating sensitive information and not sharing it with anyone. You should consider using encrypted messaging service for example, Signal or Telegram for protection of your messages from being viewed by prying eye.

Step 5: Have Backup Power

After an nuclear attack there will be power interruptions that are expected. Due to the devastation of power facilities as well as transmission cables, the electric grid could be destroyed, leaving the survivors with no light. In the absence of electricity, it would be difficult to run vital infrastructures, like water treatment facilities, hospitals as well as communications networks. In order to survive with no power, an emergency power supply plan is crucial.

The initial step to develop the backup power plan to determine your power needs. Find out what essential equipment and devices need electricity in order to operate. They could be refrigeration equipment for medical devices as well as communication equipment. When you've determined your requirements, you should consider possibilities for power backup.

The most secure alternatives for power backup is to use a diesel generator. Diesel generators are durable and run for prolonged durations, which makes them perfect for power failures that last a long time. Generators of this kind are readily available for purchase or rented through retailers of hardware or specialist dealers. Diesel generators, however, use fossil fuel and can be difficult to acquire in the post-apocalyptic future. It is best to find it at petrol stations, if you're equipped with an hazmat suit that protects from radiation. You should stockpile sufficient fuel to allow the generator to last for at minimum a few weeks.

Another option is a solar powered generator. They are lightweight simple to use and don't require energy sources. They function through harnessing sunlight with solar panels, then turning the energy into electricity before storage in batteries. Solar generators are green option, they're more prone to failure than diesel generators, and need plenty of sunshine to operate efficiently. It is therefore crucial to make sure you have enough solar panels and batteries in order to satisfy your energy needs.

Wind turbines can also be an option for back-up energy. Wind turbines of a small size are simple to set up and produce enough power to run important appliances. But, they require steady wind in order to function effectively. This can be difficult in certain regions. It is suggested to set up wind turbines in regions that have consistent winds.

In the process of developing your backup power strategy, it's important to have a reliable method of evaluating your energy consumption. This will allow you to manage the power consumption and prevent being unable to replenish your battery or fuel power in the event of an unexpected. There are a variety of instruments and gadgets for energy monitoring accessible, which range from basic power meters to sophisticated energy management tools. It is advised to select the right tool to align with the intended consumption and your budget. Make sure you monitor it frequently.

As a conclusion, having a plan for backup power is an essential element of the survival of a post nuclear world. Generators that use diesel, solar and wind turbines all are feasible choices for powering backup generators. Each has strengths and drawbacks. Therefore, it's crucial to pick which one best meets your preferences and is easiest to put in place. Be sure to track the amount of energy you use as well as stockpile sufficient battery and fuel to ensure that your backup power source operational for a long time. By preparing a backup power source will increase your odds of surviving the event of nuclear disaster.

Step 6: Practise Your Plan

Always review and test your survival plan regularly with family members. Be sure that everyone is aware of their roles and obligations when there is an emergency. Examine your emergency equipment to make sure they're useful and in good working order.

Keep in mind that the most important factor for surviving nuclear attacks is preparedness. When you develop a survival strategy together with your loved ones will help you reduce your risk and improve your chance of making it through the aftermath of a disaster.

Psychological Preparedness

The psychological aspect is as important as physical training in the event of an attack from nuclear. Following an explosion in the nuclear sector could be devastating and overwhelming However, there are steps that you can do to prepare yourself and your family emotionally in case that such a catastrophe could occur.

Learning is Key

The power of knowledge is in decreasing anxiety and taking control over a situation. Know more about the threats and hazards from a nuclear attack, along with the procedure in reducing your risk of being exposed, and boosting the chance of being able to survive. But, ensure that your sources are authentic and stay clear of sensationalized or incorrect information.

Be Realistic

It is crucial to comprehend the real-world risks associated with a nuclear strike while being mindful of the dangers of uncontrolled fear and anxiety. Consider the probabilities for the attack, which kinds of targets are the likely to be hit, and what the consequences would be. This can help keep you from making assumptions and allow you to focus on preparing for the future.

Build a Support System

It's crucial that you have a plan of defense ready before an attack with nuclear weapons occurs. Consider the possibilities of the threat with your friends and family members and establish a plan for communication in case the communication system fails. Being aware that you are surrounded by reliable sources of support during a crisis will decrease anxiety, isolation and stress.

Practise Coping Skills

Find coping strategies that you can use like exercises, meditation or simply spending time with family members, and practice them frequently. These techniques can help you reduce anxiety and stress, and ensure your safety and calm during times when you're in a state of doubt.

Build Resilience

Resilience refers to the capacity to withstand, adjust to and overcome the effects of adversity. It's an important characteristic to develop during times of stress. Take steps to build your resilience. For instance, creating healthy relationships, taking charge of your health and fitness as well as pursuing problem-solving techniques as well as developing an understanding of your the purpose and significance of your daily life.

Mental Health Support

It is not a bad idea to seek assistance with your mental health when you are feeling overwhelmed, worried or depressed over the threat of an nuclear attack. Mental health professionals will help you develop strategies for coping, go through the trauma of your past and ease anxiety.

Practise Mindfulness

It can aid you to stay focused as well as improve your capacity to make plans for the future. Consider practicing mindfulness meditation, and other methods that can aid in staying alert and sharp.

Acceptance

Acceptance refers to recognizing the realities of an event, rather than trying to avoid or deny the reality of it. Acceptance helps you to feel calm and less overwhelmed with the threat of nuclear war.

The best way to prepare psychologically for the possibility of nuclear attack requires keeping yourself informed, being honest creating a supportive system practicing coping techniques and building resilience, getting help with mental health, practicing mindfulness as well as acceptance of the circumstance. If you follow these guidelines will help you increase your mental and emotional responses to crises such as a nuclear strike.

Communication Strategy

We discussed the importance of a communications plan in the prior section.

Communication strategies are crucial when catastrophe strikes. When communications lines are cut off and it becomes difficult to contact loved ones, or reach emergency service providers It is therefore crucial to plan your strategy. These are some of the most important elements of a communications strategy in the event of an attack of nuclear nature:

Establish a Communication Chain

Find out who you must communicate with, and set up a chain using a variety of methods for contact. It could include texts, calls or emails or social media messaging applications. It is important that every person on the chain understands what they are responsible for and which ways to communicate.

Use a Designated Meeting Point

Find a place where everybody can meet. It could be your relative's residence, a communal shelter or another location that's easily accessible and safe.

Have Backup Power Sources

Make sure you are armed with backup power sources for the devices you use for communication like battery chargers for portable devices, spare batteries or even an solar-powered charger. This can help keep you active in the event of any power failure.

Practise Emergency Communication

Regularly conduct exercises with your family or group for practice in emergencies and emergency communications. This will help you identify the blind areas in your strategy and make sure everyone's comfortable with the plan.

Keep a List of Emergency Numbers

Be sure to are aware of all emergency phone numbers that include hospitals, local authorities and response services. Keep this list handy on hand, and be sure that everyone else is on an exact copy.

Filter Information

Review false data. Review unverified accounts be sure to rely only on authoritative sources for the latest information as well as specifics.

If you have a strategy for communication implemented, you will be able to remain in contact with your family and friends, as well as be informed of crucial information during an attack by nuclear. Make sure to practice your strategy often.

Off-Grid Preparedness

Preparing for the off-grid is an important part of any survival plan. Following an attack by nuclear weapons the power grids, communications networks and other systems could be destroyed or destroyed leaving those who survived with no modern amenities. In this scenario having no electricity is the best way to ensure that you're not dependent on the devices and you can support you and your family members without the need for them.

In order to increase your preparedness off grid in case of nuclear war it is essential to concentrate on three essential components: water, power and food. The power source is vital for the operation of the basic tools and equipment as well as heating your house as well as keeping in touch with the world. If you live off grid it is necessary to have alternatives to power sources like wind turbines, solar panels or generators, in order for your power needs.

Another important resource is water that is essential for living off the grid. A nuclear explosion can cause water sources to become contaminated and water treatment facilities in municipal waters could be ineffective. So, it is essential to be able to have a sustainable and reliable supply of water that is clean for your home, like a water source or rainwater harvesting system.

Food is the third essential element for living off grid. When a disaster strikes the grocery stores and supermarkets might be closed or depleted of food items. This is why you should be prepared with a stash of non-perishable foods including canned foods as well as dried fruit, in order that will last your family for a long time.

Apart from water, power as well as foods, there are many other things to think about when you are preparing for living off grid. It is essential to be equipped with basic skills for survival, like first aid, self-defense, and hunting to ensure the safety of your family and friends. Also, it is essential to prepare a strategy for sanitation, waste management as well as communication with other people.

The bottom line is that off-grid preparation is crucial to be able to withstand an attack from nuclear. Being self-sufficient, and not depending on damaged infrastructure you will be able to survive the consequences of a nuclear strike.

Below are a few actions you can follow to enhance your preparation for an off-grid emergency:

Create your own electricity by installing solar panels or wind turbines to produce your own electric power. It will provide an energy source that is reliable regardless of the power grid going down.

Secure a reliable water supply by installing rainwater collection devices or create a well so you've got a steady water source. It is also recommended to have an additional water filtering system in the event of water contamination.

Create your own food source Make a garden or greenhouse to cultivate your own food. It can provide your with fresh and well-balanced produce. It will also reduce your reliance on the supermarket shop.

Learn the essentials of survival Basic survival strategies such as fishing, hunting and food preservation, to ensure that you are able to endure an extended situation.

You should stock up on all the necessities Make sure you have a stock of the essential items you need, including water, food and first-aid supplies. Also, you should keep a backup source of fuel, including propane and wood.

Create communications lines: Create the means to talk with other people for example, satellite or ham radio. It will let you ask for help, or to gather outside data.

Make a backup plan Create a backup strategy to be prepared should your main off-grid system fails. In the event, for example, the solar panels you have are damaged or stolen, you should have the backup generator ready or other source of power.

Essential Skills

Primary

First Aid and Medical Skills

Medical facilities could be restricted or not available during an explosion of nuclear nature. This is why it's important that you have the some basic medical knowledge to deal with the effects of injuries and illnesses. Learn these skills through courses provided by organizations such as the Red Cross, local community centres, and online platforms like Coursera. In addition, it's advisable to carry a complete first-aid kit that includes essential products, including bandsages, antiseptics and painkillers.

Self-Defence and Security Skills

If you live in a post-nuclear world the safety and security of people is a major concern. Knowing self-defense and security techniques will help protect you and those around you from threats. Learn self-defense through classes in martial arts or enrolling in self-defense training courses. In addition, acquiring the basics of security including the security of your house or shed, will aid in preventing potential burglars from entering your home.

Survival Skills

The ability to survive is essential for anyone who wants to survive in the event of a disaster. Skills include constructing shelters as well as finding water that is clean as well as starting a fire as well as hunting for food. It is possible to learn survival strategies in courses run by companies such as REI or by attending outdoors survival classes. In addition, reading survival books and practicing these skills in the harsh outdoors could help.

Communication Skills

The skills of communication cannot be re-taught repeatedly enough. It is possible to learn about communication by attending radio communications or by attending seminars regarding emergency communications. In addition, it's vital to have alternative communication tools like radios that are portable, so that you are in touch with your family and friends.

Gardening and Agriculture Skills

Knowing how to garden and learn agricultural techniques is vital for self-sufficiency. The skills required include the planting of and maintaining the crops and cultivating animals. It is possible to learn the basics of agriculture and gardening through courses provided by local agricultural centers or at community gardens. Also, practicing these techniques within your own backyard or your community garden could give you practical experience.

Tinkering Skills

Engineering and mechanical skills can be crucial for fixing or making repairs to essential equipment, including vehicles, generators, and other equipment. Learn these abilities through courses in basic mechanical repairs, or taking part in workshops for small engine maintenance. In addition, practicing the basics of repairs for your personal vehicles and equipment could help you develop knowledge.

It's important to keep in mind that, while you may not require all the skills in the immediate future, spending time studying them could assist you in adjusting to the new challenges that come with an era post-nuclear.

Secondary

Bartering and Negotiation Skills

Bartering is a method of swap of products or services that do not require the use of currency and negotiation is the process of coming to an agreement via discussions and compromise. For a better understanding of the art of bartering and negotiation begin by understanding the significance of different products and services when you are in a scenario. It is also important to practice communication and interpersonal abilities, along with negotiation strategies that include compromise as well as win-win strategies. Try practicing with your friends and relatives by trading items or services as well as making a fair trade.

Leadership and Teamwork Skills

Teamwork and leadership skills are essential for a successful emergency response and survival even after the nuclear threat. In times of crisis, efficient leadership and teamwork are essential. In order to master these abilities it is important to begin building strong communication skills and the capacity to effectively delegate work. It is also possible to develop connections and trust with other people and also develop skills in problem solving and decision making. You might consider joining a local group or a course in leadership for knowledge in these fields.

Chapter 10: Home Defence--Securing Your Property And Staying Safe

In the event of a crisis you can turn your house into your castle. It is crucial to protect your house and guard your perimeter from outside threats. Security for your home isn't the simple matter of having a solid doors and locks. You need a plan of action and the appropriate tools as well as a thorough knowledge of how to utilize these tools. The chapter below will provide strategies for protecting your property and remaining safe during the case an attack from nuclear. From securing your home, and establishing a strong defense plan, we'll examine practical and reliable methods to safeguard your family from the threat lurking around.

Identifying Potential Weaknesses

One of the first steps to improve the security of your home is to recognize its vulnerabilities. Start by looking over your house's borders, and looking for places that are easily attacked by a burglar. Think about factors such as the fence's height as well as the state of your gates, as well as the security of the locks. Check for areas within your property which provide security for the intruder or serve to hide. Within your home, check the state of the windows and doors Consider any possible areas of intrusion. After you've identified the areas of concern, you are able to make steps to strengthen and ensure their security.

Reinforcing Doors and Windows

Windows and doors are among the primary entrance points for burglars therefore it's important to strengthen them in order to stop the entry of intruders who are not authorized. Think about replacing weak doors or frames with more durable material, like solid timber or steel. Install security plates and deadbolts to stop doors from being smashed. Windows can be secured with steel grilles and security films. Also, it is important to lock windows whenever they are not being used.

Installing a Home Security System

A home security system acts as a security measure and deterrent against potential burglars. The system will contain sensors at windows and doors along with motion detectors as well as security cameras. Modern systems are remotely monitored, and alert you as well as the authorities of an incident. You should consider installing an siren or alarm to notify your neighbors and you should there be a burglary.

Creating a Safe Room

In the event of an incident, an safe room could provide an enclave in which you can hide. It is possible to create a safe space could be a room that has strong walls, and an locked door. It could be an existing area in your house which is modified using the proper security measures. It should be equipped with the ability to use a cell phone or other communication device as well as a first-aid kit, self-defense weapons and other supplies that will last for at least a couple of months.

Acquiring Defensive Equipment

A variety of defensive gear on hand could provide another security layer. These include products like pepper spray Tasers, as well as firearms. But, it's important to adhere to all local law and regulations in the case of owning or using weapons for defense.

Establishing a Neighbourhood Watch Program

A neighborhood watch program will assist in preventing potential criminals from entering your property and provide safety for the community. Collaborate with neighbors to develop a system with regular patrols and notifications. Through observing one another and reporting suspicious activities and responsibilities, you will create an atmosphere that is safe for everyone.

Creating an Emergency Response Plan

The existence of a strategy in case of emergencies could help you react rapidly and effectively. Your plan should provide directions on how to reach emergency services, a specific location for family members to meet and a procedure to follow in an the event of an emergency. Be sure that the members of the family are aware and can access the document.

Practising Home Defence Drills

Constantly practicing home defence drills will help you prepare to tackle a crisis without flinching. It could include the practice of trails for evacuation routes, undertaking drills for fire, as well as practicing using defensive gear.

Evacuation and Escape Planning

In certain situations the need may arise to leave your house. Be sure all members of your family are aware of the evacuation route and that they have a specific location outside the house for a meeting. It's also essential to create a plan in your home for pets as well as other essentials that require to be transported to the emergency room.

Chapter 11: Stockpiling

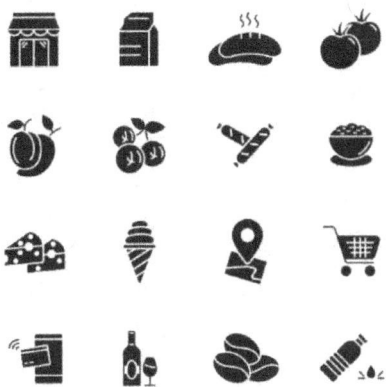

If you find yourself in emergency, if you have an adequately-stocked pantry as well as an emergency kit of supplies You can avoid desperation. Storing involves an accumulation of vital products, items as well as provisions that will help you and your family throughout a range of crisis situations, such as natural catastrophes, economic collapse and social unrest. A well-stocked pantry and emergency supplies kit provides you up with all the necessities that you require when searching to find them isn't an alternative.

In this section we'll go over the essentials of stockpiling. We'll cover which items to put in stockpiles in the first place, the amount to store as well as where you can store your items. In addition, we'll discuss the necessity of rotating your items and ways to ensure that your stocks are maintained throughout time. When you're done with this section, you'll be equipped with a an understanding of how to maintain and build an adequate stockpile of supplies that will aid you in surviving even the most difficult of situations.

Food and Water Supplies

Food access will be extremely limited after the nuclear explosion. Food stores will become empty and supply chains could be interrupted. It is crucial to keep a supply of non-perishable foods in order to survive the aftermath of an attack. This guide will provide suggestions on what types of foods to store and their importance in terms of nutrition and the necessary quantities that two people will need to last for 14 days.

In the first place, it is important to choose food items that have high nutritional value and that have a long time to shelf. This includes canned fruits and veggies, dry fruit as well as beans, nuts, pasta, rice peanut butter, pasta, crackers. They are rich in proteins, carbohydrates, as well as important minerals and vitamins. Contained stews and soups are an good sources of nutrition and are able to be eaten with no cooking or heating.

It is essential to have a sufficient quantity of water available in addition. The standard rule is to keep one gallon of water for each person each day. The amount you need may differ according to individual preferences as well as the climate of the area you live in. It is suggested to keep at minimum 2 weeks' worth water available.

To determine the amount of food items to store, take into account the energy requirements of every person. A typical adult needs between 2,200 to 2,500 calories a day. For two individuals to last for 14 days one day, it's necessary to store between 56,000 and 75,000 calories worth of food items.

To make sure you've got sufficient nutritional diversity within your food In order to ensure that you have enough variety in your diet, keep a stockpile of a mixture of protein along with carbohydrates, fats, and. Tuna cans, chicken as well as beef jerky, are all excellent sources of protein. Likewise, rice, pasta, as well as crackers provide carbs. Nuts and peanut butter are rich in good fats that are able to provide more calories.

It's also crucial to think about the methods of preparation that you will need for the food items you have in your pantry. There is a good chance that power is not working and gas lines are snared. Thus, you should stockpile food items which can be eaten without heating or cooking. Snacks and meals that can be eaten immediately can be a great choice in this scenario.

In the end, it's essential to rotate regularly your food storage containers to make sure that the food does not get rotten. Most non-perishable foods are able to last for a long time However, eventually they'll end up expiring. You should check the expiration dates on your food at least every 6 months, and then rotate products that have expired out.

A well-stocked pantry is an essential part of a nuclear survival strategy. The importance of focusing on high-nutrition items that last a long time will guarantee that you're equipped with enough food to last. Make sure you have enough water in your stockpile and think about the calories for each of members.

According to the food stockpiling guide, this shopping list of items is recommended for 2 persons to be able to live for 14 days

canned meats (tuna and salmon, chicken, etc.) 14 cans

Canned fruit and vegetables Cans of 28

Peanut butter or another peanut butter 1 big Jar

Rice cakes or crackers four boxes

Cereal bars, or granola bars 14 bars

Dried fruits and nuts: two large bags

Pasta or rice 4 bags

Chilli soup canned in cans or soup 14 cans

Shelf-stable milk (cow milk, soy milk, etc.) 4 cartons

Water: 28 gallons / 127L (or 1 gallon / 4.5L per person per day)

It is vital to keep in mind that this is an general outline and the actual amount and type of foods may differ based on your personal diet preferences, restrictions and personal preference. Make sure to regularly check and rotate your foodstuffs to ensure the foods you have in your pantry are safe in terms of consumption over a longer time.

Other than food Other items suggested to be part of the nuclear kit are:

A water filtration system, or tablets

First aid kit

Flashlights, lanterns or flashlights equipped with additional batteries

Portable radio that comes with additional batteries

Basic toiletries (toothbrush, toothpaste, soap, etc.)

Disposable cups, plates and kitchen dishes

Can opener

Garbage bags

Blankets, or sleeping bags

Wear warm clothing

Shoes that are sturdy

The food and water instructions will help you navigate safely through a nuclear disaster.

Medical Supplies

Medical equipment is required to treat physical ailments however, medical supplies and knowledge could be deficient or not available in the event of a nuclear crisis. This is why it's essential to have a supply of essential medical items as well as learn the basics of first aid to improve our odds of being able to survive.

In the first place, it's vital to have an extensive first aid kit in your arsenal. It should contain basic medical items, like gauze, bandages and antiseptics as well as scissors and tape. In addition, it is worth adding over-the-counter medications to treat pain as well as fever control, among other ailments that are common. It is recommended to have enough stockpiled that last for at least 2 weeks after the strike.

In the event of radiation exposure in the body, potassium Iodide (KI) could be the lifesaver. It protects the thyroid gland from the effects of radioactive iodine. This can result in thyroid cancer. It's best to buy sufficient KI tablets to cover all family members.

Damages caused by blasts including burns fractures, and cuts may require specialized medical treatment. Store items such as splints wound irrigation systems, as well as burn-related dressings within your inventory. Also, you should consider storing an essential surgical kit which includes sterile sutures, gloves and scalpels.

Alongside physical injuries Mental health too can be impacted. Therapies such as anti-anxiety drugs and sedatives are a great way to deal with anxiety and stress. Prepare a record of prescribed medications every family member might require since the availability of pharmacies could be restricted.

It's vital to keep in mind that, while storing medical supplies is essential in the preparations for a nuclear attack It's also important to master the basics of medical knowledge. Learning a course in first aid and knowing how to treat commonly-occurring injuries and illnesses could be a huge help when faced with an crisis. Furthermore, being able to recognize and treat radiation-related illnesses should be considered seriously due to the reason in that.

Information on medical stockpiling sources are those from the Red Cross, the Centers for Disease Control and Prevention (CDC) as well as FEMA. Additionally, there are a variety of websites and books available that can help you learn more.

Here's a list of items to buy of medical supplies recommended to be prepared for a post nuclear strike emergency:

Adhesive bandages (assorted sizes)

Gauze pads (assorted sizes)

Sterile gauze rolls

Medical tape

Wipes or antiseptic solutions

Potassium Iodide (KI) Tablets

Antibiotic ointment

Hydrogen peroxide

Handsanitizer based on alcohol

Pain relief medication (acetaminophen, ibuprofen, aspirin)

Anti-diarrhoea medication

Anti-nausea medication

Antihistamine medication

Prescription medication (if necessary)

Tweezers

Scissors

Thermometer

Nitrile or latex gloves

Face masks

Eye eye protection

Sterile Saline Solution

The first aid manual

The Survival Manual (including medical emergency)

The medical reference guide (with dosage guidelines and instructions for use)

Trauma kit (including tourniquets compress bandages, tourniquet chest seals)

Kit for Surgical (including scalpel, forceps as well as surgical scissors)

Quickly clotting powder, or gauze

IV fluids and tubing

IV administration kit

Blood pressure cuff, Stethoscope

-Splint as well as other devices for immobilisation

The list of inventory items is dependent on the quantity of people you're stocking for, as well as the duration of time you're hoping to remain protected. Make sure to check expiration dates frequently and change items as necessary to guarantee their efficiency in the event of an situation of emergency.

Defensive Equipment and Tools

Although many survival guides concentrate on the need for food and medical equipment defense equipment to protect and self-defense deserve the same importance. In this article we'll explore diverse kinds of weapons, protection equipment and the tools required to survive an area that has been irradiated.

Protective Gear

A proper protective equipment is essential to protect yourself from physical harms. A gas mask is an ideal first step however, it's essential that you wear a full body suit that protects against radiation exposure. Plastic or rubber are suggested together with gloves and boots that prevent the skin from contact with any radiation-producing materials. The suits can be purchased through various online retailers and are also available in large quantities for groups of larger sizes.

Weapons

It is common for people to be forced to follow every-man-for-his own-way of life in crisis deadlocks. This is why it's important to carry guns for self-defense as well as for protection of your possessions. Guns that include shotguns, rifles, or handguns are highly recommended together with an adequate quantity of ammunition. Also, it is recommended to carry melee weapons like clubs and knives that are suitable for close-quarter battle. They can be purchased from licensed dealers or online retailers.

Tools for Building and Repairing Structures

The ability to construct or fix structures in order to provide shelter and security. This is why it's vital to have the proper tools to accomplish these jobs. The basic toolkit must include saws, hammers and screwscrewdrivers, pliers and wrenches. Additionally, an assortment of screws, nails as well as other fasteners is necessary. The tools are available at hardware stores or on-line retailers.

Conclusion

If you stock up on safety tools, equipment as well as tools for building or repairing structures, you'll improve your odds for survival in a post-nuclear world. Be sure to buy these products from reliable suppliers, and be sure to follow the safety rules in using the items. Keep safe and always be ready.

Bartering and Trade Supplies

If the situation is dire, circumstances, trade and bartering could become commonplace. The possession of items that can be traded like toiletries, food items, clothing, is crucial in ensuring accessibility to the other essential things. Cash in the form of a stash and other items of value can also be utilized to bartering or trade.

Here are a few suggestions to items that could be utilized to barter post nuclear strike

Towels: in a future that is without water, the most basic sanitation items are extremely sought after. Soap, toothpaste, toothbrushes shampoo, as well as other toiletries could be utilized to exchange currency.

The clothing: Clothes are an important item that is very popular. You should consider stocking up on extra clothing like warmer coats and hats and gloves, and tough boots.

Food that is Non-Perishable: Food things, like dried fruit, canned foods such as nuts, jerky, and other snacks are valuable in the post nuclear world. You should ensure that you have sufficient food items for your loved ones, and think about keeping some extra food items for trade.

Medical Treatment: Prescription drugs can be an asset to those suffering from chronic illness. Make sure you have enough medication in your stock to combat chronic or recurring diseases.

Tools: In a world with decimated infrastructure, construction/engineering tools will be a desired commodity. Tools for hand like saws, hammers, shovels and axes are going to prove useful in restoring houses and other buildings.

Fuel: Propane, gasoline and various other fuels are in short supply therefore, making them essential. Keep a stockpile of extra fuel whenever you can, since it could be used to power vehicles, generators as well as other equipment.

Water: Although it's important to keep a reserve of water for your family members, additional water is a good option as bartering. Think about investing in a filtering system, or collect extra water bottles.

Seeds: When people start in rebuilding their lives they'll have to start growing the food they consume. The seeds that are stored for fruit such as vegetables and grains is a good purchase for the possibility of bartering.

Important to keep in mind the fact that these suggestions are only general suggestions and should be adapted to your particular situation. Think about your home's location, family's size and the possibility of bartering partners before deciding on which things to store.

To track the inventory in your warehouse, make an inventory spreadsheet and periodically make it updated. The supplies you have should be organized and readily accessible to authorized members.

Sanitation and Hygiene Supplies

Water and food won't be enough to ensure your life when a disease strikes you in the first place. A clean and healthy environment can prevent you from this potentially life-threatening condition. In this article we'll go over the most essential items you'll should have in your arsenal to ensure your home and surroundings spotless as well as your family safe.

The very first thing you'll need is a source of water. Although you'll need another supply of water for drinking as well, you'll need water to wash your hands. Make sure you have at least 1 gallon of water per individual each day to wash and cleaning. In addition, put in filters for water in your shelter, like an aeration-based filter or a ceramic filter to make sure there is a constant source of water that is clean.

The next step is to have the soap you've bought and cleaners. Try to find a mixture of liquid soap, bar soap and hand sanitizers with antibacterial properties to ensure that you have everything covered for hygiene. Also, you'll need lots of cleaning products including bleach, sprays for disinfectants and antiseptic wipes, in order to cleanse surfaces and wash equipment.

What's the reason you shouldn't have sparkling teeth when you're that has been blown up to size? The personal hygiene products are vital for survival post-nuclear.

Get toothbrushes, toothpaste, floss, and mouthwashes for maintaining dental hygiene. If you want to bathe, think about buying body wash, dry shampoo with no rinse cleansing foams. Baby wipes are an option for sensitive skin that could be used to clean yourself, as well as equipment and surfaces.

Toilet facilities might not be available following a nuclear attack and it's essential to keep a amount of hygiene items. Disposable pads and disposable diapers are a great option for multiple uses for example, as bandages that can be made up or alternatives to toilet paper. Additionally, keep a stockpile of litter bags, garbage bags litter and sawdust to make an impromptu toilet. You might consider buying a camper's portable toilet, or even a bucket that has toilet seats for more comfort and cleanliness.

Concerning medical supplies you should stockpile essential items for first aid, like gauze, bandages as well as antiseptic Ointments. Additionally, you should keep an inventory of latex gloves as well as face masks for protection against disease and infection. Razors for disposal and nail clippers are also helpful tools for maintaining your personal hygiene, and to prevent infection.

The bottom line is that proper hygiene and sanitation are essential aspects for survival in the post-apocalyptic era. The stockpile of soap, water, products for cleaning and personal hygiene products as well as sanitation supplies will help keep your home clean and hygienic living space. The goal is not only to survive but to thrive during a disaster. Make sure you take care of your hygiene and remain well.

Here's a complete guide to the most essential hygiene and sanitation supplies to keep in your stockpile post nuclear strike

Bleach: for sanitizing areas and sources of water 1 gallon for each person over a period of two weeks.

soap: to wash hands and general hygiene. Three bars for each person over the duration of two weeks.

Tobacco and toothpaste to ensure oral hygiene. Two tubes of toothpaste as well as two toothbrushes each for a 2-week time.

Toilet paper for individual hygiene and sanitation. 30 rolls per person over the duration of two weeks.

The products are designed for feminine hygiene to help women maintain their personal hygiene. One box for each woman over a period of two weeks.

Disposable diapers, wipes and disposables used for hygiene at the infant level 2 diapers, and two wipes for each infant over a period of two weeks.

Disposable gloves used to clean up contaminated substances Two boxes per individual for the duration of two weeks.

Hand sanitizer for hands hygiene if water and soap are not readily available. Three bottles per user for the duration of two weeks.

Trash bags to dispose of waste that is contaminated and trash. 10 bags of large size per household for a 2 week time.

The list below isn't exhaustive and the amount you need will vary based on the size of your home and the amount of time you're planning to remain secure. Also, it is recommended to place these things in a cool, dry and dark area so that they can last longer.

The best sources of information to prepare this equipment are the The CDC's Emergency Preparedness and Response website as well as the FEMA's Ready.gov website. In addition local emergency management organizations and organizations for disaster relief might provide advice and assistance that are specific to the location you live in.

Fuel and Energy Supplies

Imagine a scenario in which power grids have gone down and conventional energy sources are no anymore accessible. In times of crisis having access to energy as well as energy is crucial.

The initial step to gather sources of energy and fuel is determining your requirements. What is the minimum time you'll need to live without conventional sources of energy? One week? Two weeks? One month? The longer you'll need to live, the greater amount of fuel and energy sources you will require.

One of the primary kinds of fuels to store is gasoline. The fuel is vital for the powering of motors and generators and can prove invaluable in a post nuclear strike environment. If you are planning to store gasoline, it is essential to pick the correct containers. Containers made of metal are the ideal option as they're more resistant to leaks and are able to withstand temperatures that can be extreme.

Propane is a different fuel that you should consider. It is a fuel that can be utilized for heating, cooking even for lighting. If you are planning to stockpile propane, be sure to take into consideration the types of appliances which use propane, and then calculate the amount it will take to run them to the required time.

Apart from propane and gasoline, you should consider different types of fuel including coal, firewood or charcoal. They can be utilized to cook food, heat and for lighting. The firewood must be kept in a well-ventilated, dry space to avoid rot and humidity.

Solar energy is an excellent alternative to conventional sources of power and is used for powering lights, small appliances and a generator. In order to build up solar power devices is important to select the best solar panels and charge controllers and batteries that are able to withstand high temperatures as well as provide steady energy.

The wind power source is another alternative to harness to generate energy. Small wind turbines can be utilized to produce electric power, and then stored in batteries to be later used. usage.

As well as supply of energy or fuel You must also have tools for maintaining the machine that generates energy or uses it. These include items like the spark plug, filters for oil and wrenches.

Here are a few items to consider as well as the quantity needed by two persons to last for 2 weeks:

Gasoline: 30 gallons

Propane: 4-6 20lb tanks

Portable generator

Charcoal: 20 lbs

Firewood: 30-40 wood

Batteries: 30-40 each (AA AAA, AA and D)

Solar panels: 3 small, portable panels

A solar-powered battery charger

Flashlights

Candles

Oil lamps

Spark plugs

Oil filters

Wrenches

The gasoline is used to power transport, generators, as well as cooking when needed. Propane is great to cook with and is also a great option to heat your home if you own an propane heater. The firewood and charcoal can be used to cook with and additionally provide warmth. Batteries are vital to power radios, flashlights as well as other electronic gadgets. Solar panels are a great way to recharge batteries and devices throughout the day.

Be sure to keep all energy and fuel supplies in a dry, cool and ventilated area, free of source of heat or flame. Be sure you possess the tools and equipment required to deal with and store the fuel.

Clothing and Protective Gear

After the nuclear explosion can make victims vulnerable to a myriad of risks, such as exposure to radiation as well as harsh environment conditions. To ensure your safety and wellbeing It is vital to wear appropriate clothing and safety equipment.

In selecting clothes to wear in a post nuclear world it is crucial to pick clothes that are sturdy and useful. The clothes you choose to wear will shield you from elements as well as the risks of radiation exposure. Find fabrics which are strong and tight-woven, such as canvas or denim as they provide an effective shield from radioactive particles.

As well as the protective clothes, you'll also require personal protection apparatus (PPE) to protect your body from hazards of the environment. It could include things like respirators and gloves, as well as helmets as well as goggles. The importance of respirators is in protecting against the inhalation radioactive substances, whereas gloves and goggles protect your eyes and hands from germs and contaminated surfaces.

You should have enough clothing sets for everyone in your family. The best rule of thumb is to own at minimum two sets of clothes per person, together with a complete package of PPE.

The other things to think about adding to your clothes and protective gear stash include:

Rubber boots: They are a great way to shield your feet from the contaminating surface and ground.

Rain gear will help you stay warm and dry in cold winter conditions.

Duct tape: This flexible tool can be utilized to close gaps in garments and equipment.

Keep in mind that radiation exposure poses the greatest threat for survival in a post-nuclear future therefore it is crucial to implement precautions to avoid exposure.

The best sources of information on selecting and buying protective clothing and equipment are government websites as well as store selling safety equipment. Do not be hesitant to seek guidance from professionals in the area, and make sure you test the equipment prior to use outdoors.

Make your time to do your research and purchase quality products ensure there is enough food for everyone within your family.

Here's a suggestion for a listing of gear that is recommended in order to allow two persons to live for the duration of two weeks:

Four pairs of durable hiking boots, work boots, or other shoes

8 pairs of thick socks

Four pairs of tough work gloves

Two pairs of chemical resistant gloves

Two pairs of safety goggles

Two full-face respirator masks, with spare cartridges

8 N95 respirator face masks

8 disposable gloves

8 disposable coveralls

16 dust masks

Four Sets of rain-gear (jacket and trousers)

8 sets of thermal underwear (shirt and pant)

8 pairs of cozy socks

8 warm hats

Eight pairs of gloves that are insulated or mittens

8 winter jackets and coats

8 pairs of glasses

Note that this is only a general suggestion of quantity and could vary depending upon your personal situation. Always make sure to assess the needs of your family and modify in accordance with your own needs.

Communication and Technology Supplies

In the absence of functioning devices for communication and technologies, survivors of nuclear accidents will remain in a state of isolation and vulnerability. In this article we'll look at the most essential technology and communication equipment that survivors must be equipped with.

In the first place, it's essential to be able to rely on a reliable method for communications. It could be walkie-talkies and two-way radios as well as radios with ham codes. Two-way radios make a fantastic alternative for communication in short ranges as ham radios provide longer-range communications and have accessibility to the emergency channels. Make sure you have spare batteries in order to run these radios for a long time.

Also, you must be able to recharge the devices used for communication. Portable solar powered chargers are an ideal choice since it recharges with the sun and is able to charge gadgets like smartphones, tablets as well as laptops. A power bank spare or battery powered charger can come useful on days of rain and other unforeseen situations.

Being able to access real-time updates and data is a must. A portable AM/FM radio with the ability to get emergency updates and broadcasts is an essential. Hand-cranked or solar-powered radio is a great choice since it doesn't require power to function.

A third important element of communications as well as technology concerns lighting. Set up a mixture of battery powered or solar-powered lighting, such as lanterns, flashlights and headlamps. They'll provide perfect lighting for navigation and for carrying out important tasks like cooking or reading.

In the end, you should be prepared to safeguard the security of your communications as well as technology equipment. Get a container that is waterproof for protecting electronics from water as well as a Faraday bag that protects the devices from EMP.

Make sure you have enough food and other items to provide at least two weeks of living to two people. Be sure to regularly check and keep up-to-date your communication and tech supplies to make sure that they are operational.

This is a shopping list of items recommended and gadgets to last two weeks of desperation for two persons:

Portable two-way radios with portable transmitters 4 (2 per individual)

Hand-cranked, solar-powered or emergency radio 1

Batteries spare for all electronic devices when necessary

Satellite phone: 1 (optional however strongly advised)

Tablet or laptop equipped with survival guides pre-installed and maps.

Map and Compass 1 set

Solar-powered or battery-powered lights Three of each

Container with waterproofing 1

Faraday bag 1

Lockable storage container 1

The amount of equipment required will vary based on your personal preference and budget. However, the checklist can provide an ideal start for two persons who want to make sure they have reliable communication and accessibility to technology following an attack on nuclear power.

Take care when storing the gadgets. Choose a dry, secure area and regularly check to see if the device functions and how long it has been in use.

In accumulating these communications and technological supplies, families as well as families are able to improve coordination between them after the nuclear crisis.

Recreational Supplies

The world as we understand could alter in a moment. If there is a nuclear attack and a catastrophic event, survival is the primary goal. In addition to ensuring you have access things, like water, food, and medical aids, are vital, it's also crucial to think about the mental and emotional health of your family when dealing with the aftermath of a catastrophe. That's where your leisure and entertainment items come in.

Be prepared for the psychological strain from a nuclear attack to be massive. The survivors may be feeling isolated or anxious. They may also feel feeling overwhelmed by the loss their old life. These are difficult times and the pursuit of entertainment and recreation are a crucial factor in helping families and individuals maintain their emotional and psychological wellbeing.

An organized recreational kit could provide an important distraction as well as aid in keeping people entertained throughout long stretches of sitting. These are the things to think about when designing your recreational kit

Magazines and books The availability of magazines and books can aid in keeping your mind active and provide an opportunity to escape real life.

Puzzles and board games Games and puzzles on the board can be fun, but they can also help develop critical thinking and thinking skills for problem solving. They are a fantastic opportunity to spend time with your the family and your colleagues.

The game of playing cards: A deck of cards could provide unending entertainment and could are suitable for playing a wide range of games.

Instruments for music If you or someone in your family is a musician, you should think of having a small instrument such as the harmonium or the ukulele.

Art equipment Art supplies: Drawing and painting may be therapeutic ways to release emotions and reduce anxiety. You should consider including crayons with different colors, a sketchpad along with brushes and paints to your art kit.

Sport equipment: Exercising is vital to maintain of both mental and physical well-being. You should think about adding items such as the frisbee, a jump rope or a ball in an exciting game of catch.

Electronics: Though electric power may be limited following the impact of nuclear war however, having a radio and handheld gaming console will help keep you entertained for a long time as well as provide an interface with the outside world.

Apart from the points that are mentioned earlier, it's crucial to also consider the storage and security of entertainment and leisure equipment. An outdoor container is able to safeguard your items from being damaged and a locking storage container will help keep your items safe from loss or theft.

Keep in mind that even though survival post-nuclear is the main concern wellbeing of the mind and body is a prerequisite for living a full and productive life. Incorporating recreational products into the emergency kit could provide the sense of peace as well as a necessary break during an otherwise challenging time.

Chapter 12: Warning And Communication

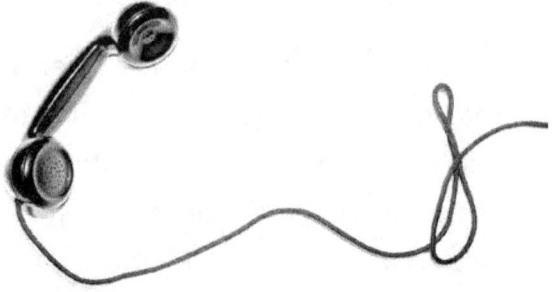

When you are in a crisis in times of crisis, having the right information is essential to survival. In order to survive and effectively, it's important to be smart when you take your next step. This is the reason using a dependable system to receive warnings and communicate to others is vital for anyone who is a survivalist or a prepper.

In this section we'll look at the different methods for understanding and responding to emergency alerts that include weather warnings, as well as civil defence alerts. We will also examine ways of establishing an effective way of communicating with your family members or friends as well as others within your local community. The chapter will also discuss fundamental communication techniques and protocols to use for a range of emergencies. No matter if you're facing an natural catastrophe or a human-made disaster, being aware and being able to communicate will ensure that you are and those you love safe.

Types of Warnings: Early Warning Systems and Alerts

The early warning systems are created to identify potential dangers and provide prior warnings to citizens as well as communities so that they can prepare and make the necessary preparations. The systems may include technology like seismic monitors, meteorological satellites, as well as chemical sensors. Seismic monitors are instruments that are used to measure and detect the seismic activity of crust of the Earth, produced by tectonic plate movements and various geological phenomena. These monitors can assist in the detection and study earthquakes, determine their probability as well as provide an early warning system to populations at risk of earthquakes. Seismic monitors employ a variety of techniques, such as accelerometers and seismometers to identify and quantify the power and frequency of earthquake waves.

Spacecrafts equipped with instruments that are designed to monitor and assess the earth's atmosphere, oceans and the land surface. They are able to provide live information about conditions in the weather, like temperatures, cloud cover, precipitation, as well as atmospheric pressure. These data are used to make forecasts for weather as well as monitor weather patterns and natural catastrophes like tornadoes, hurricanes and flooding.

Chemical sensors can be used to measure and detect the amount of chemical compounds in the atmosphere, water or even in the soil. They're able to detect and monitor various compounds, which include gasses, pollutants, as well as toxic substances. Chemical sensors are extensively used in mining, manufacturing, agriculture. They also play a role for environmental monitoring and emergency response. They are able to detect the presence of chemical spills, leaks, assess the air quality and determine the presence of harmful chemicals in the air.

Furthermore, alerts are sent via text message, or via email, to ensure that the people get timely alerts of threat that is imminent.

The Role of Emergency Broadcasts in Communication

In times of emergency the broadcasts of radio and television can be crucial to reach a large number of individuals in a brief period of time. The broadcasts of emergency situations could provide important information like the nature of danger, evacuation directions as well as safety guidelines. It is crucial for everyone to be able to access an electric or battery-powered radio in order to be able to hear emergency announcements especially in the event of power failures are experienced.

The Power of Social Media in Disseminating Warnings

Social media platforms have evolved into essential tools to disseminate crucial information and alerts in crises. Platforms such as Twitter, Facebook, and Instagram are able for sharing information, provide instructions, and respond to questions of those who are affected by the crisis. It is crucial to check the legitimacy of information posted via social media prior to making any decisions based on it.

The Role of Emergency Services in Communication

In times of emergency, the responder service including policemen or firemen have a vital role in distributing information to people and their communities. The emergency services provide information on the current situation or distribute aid and supplies. They also ensure evacuations in the affected regions. It is crucial for everyone to adhere to the guidelines of emergency personnel in an emergency situation for their safety.

The Role of Technology in Warnings and Communication

Technology advancements have dramatically changed the method by which warnings and details are communicated during emergencies. Social media apps, mobile applications as well as other platforms have been a valuable tool for emergency service personnel to connect with people. It is nevertheless essential to have backup communications methods to use in the event that technology fails.

The Future of Warnings and Communication

With technology continuing to develop as it does, the nature of warnings and communications in emergency situations is expected to shift too. Emerging technologies, including drones, artificial Intelligence, as well as smart home devices are already in use for the management of disasters and response.

Drones

One of the main purposes of drones in the scenario described above is to provide an alternative method of monitoring the areas affected by the attack. The drones could help authorities evaluate the damages, locate regions of high radiation as well as locate victims and survivors without placing emergency personnel at danger. Drones can also have sensors that determine the amount of radiation to determine the severity of impact. Drones can also be utilized for transporting medical supplies or food items, as well as water to people in need. When infrastructure is broken or destroyed this could make it difficult to get these items using traditional methods. But drones can help to move these essential items swiftly and effectively. Additionally, they could be utilized for transporting medical professionals and others first responders to zones affected by the attack, and bypass obstacles including radiation, debris, or other obstructions. A different possible use for drones following an attack by nuclear weapons would be as a search and rescue mission.

Drones by thermal cameras or other sensors are able to identify survivors in amidst of the debris, or in locations where conventional rescue methods are dangerous due to the high level of radiation. Drones with thermal imaging cameras can quickly traverse large areas and pinpoint areas where people may require rescue. Drones may also be employed to track the movements of individuals who are in the area affected. This can be helpful to stop the spread of disease by making sure that the affected population is not traveling with high levels radiation. In addition, drones can assist in enforcing the quarantine procedures or to identify people with signs of radiation illness. In addition, drones may serve for provide the possibility of communicating in regions where conventional communications infrastructure has been destroyed or removed. Drones with communications equipment can function as a portable communications hub which allows those within the affected region to connect with family members, emergency services as well as any other support networks.

There is no doubt that drones following an nuclear strike could play a crucial function in various tasks, ranging from assessing the affected area, assessing damages to providing essential supplies and facilitating communicating. While drone technology continues to advance and develop in the future, the possible applications of drones in disaster mitigation and recovery will continue to grow. It is crucial to keep in mind that the use of drones for this purpose requires cautious planning and coordination for ensuring that they're employed safely and efficiently.

Artificial Intelligence

AI is rapidly evolving technology, which is currently utilized in a variety of areas, such as security and defence. If it is the threat of nuclear war, AI could help in many ways, like earlier detection of radiation level changes, planning for response, and even recovery strategies.

One of the key benefits of AI during the time of an attack on nuclear material is the early detection. Artificial intelligence-powered sensors and devices are able to detect radiation levels as well as other indications of nuclear explosions which allows authorities to swiftly react and provide adequate warnings to the people. Furthermore, AI could be used to check social media sites and other information sources for indications of a possible attack. It can also provide an immediate alert system to help in the evacuation process.

AI may have a significant role in the planning of a response. In the event of a nuclear strike it would take an enormous amount of information to be processed, including data regarding the position of the zero point, the severity of damage in terms of radiation levels, as well as the condition of emergency aid. AI technology could to process the data in a speedy manner and provide emergency personnel with live details about the current situation helping them make better well-informed decisions and to respond efficiently.

Following an attack on nuclear weapons, AI could be used to aid in the recovery process. Artificial intelligence-powered robots can be employed to examine and clean debris, locate and identify survivors and help emergency responders in implementing rescue methods. In addition, AI can aid in tracking and oversee allocation of aids as well as first aid. This will ensure they reach those who require they most.

The deployment of AI during the case of nuclear attacks can also have an important effect on the safety of people. AI-based systems can be employed to analyze data regarding the spreading of radiation as well as other toxic substances, aiding in the process of helping find safe zones that people can leave to. AI can also be employed to facilitate evacuation to ensure that individuals are completely evacuated and are properly accounted for.

But, it's important to keep in mind that the application of AI does not come without problems. AI systems can be complicated and take a lot of resources to develop and keep them up to date. Also, they run the risk of false positives or false negatives that could result in incorrect decisions. In addition, there are ethical issues regarding AI for security and defence actions, specifically in the areas such as autonomous weapons technology.

In short, the application of AI during the case of nuclear attacks can have an effect on the early detection of a nuclear attack as well as response planning and recovery strategies. The use of AI for security and defence has its own challenges as well, so careful consideration should be paid to the ethical implications employing these tools when it comes to this.

Smart Home Devices

Smart home appliances have become more and more popular over the past few time, giving homeowners the most enthralling level of comfort in controlling their home. What happens if we don't have the possibility of a nuclear attack? Could these gadgets be of use in the future?

It's a fact. Smart home appliances can be a major factor in increasing the protection of homes and preparing in case of nuclear strike. The devices make use of a variety of sensors, cameras, as well as communications technologies that allow homeowners to control and monitor different aspects of their home from a distance, and provide real-time data and alerts.

Homeowners can secure their properties remotely can simplify security strategies. A lot of smart home appliances come equipped with cameras which can be connected to an iPhone or another similar device. This could be particularly useful in the case of nuclear strike, when there is a chance that it's not safe for people to leave the house to inspect the house. Owners of homes can make use of cameras to watch the outside of their houses and get alerted about unusual activities. Additionally, they can use smart locks that lock and open doors from afar, providing another layer of security.

Smart home appliances can be employed to regulate energy consumption in the event in the event of nuclear war. Smart thermostats are used by homeowners to regulate temperatures in their residences remotely, which will ensure an optimum temperature and reducing energy. Smart lighting systems may also be used to control the light on and off from a distance to create the illusion of there is someone at home, which can discourage potential burglars.

In addition, smart home appliances are a great way to communicate when there is a nuclear threat. There are many devices that come equipped with microphones and speakers which are used to talk to family members, or even emergency assistance. Owners of homes can use smart speakers to get emergencies alerts as well as broadcasts and keep them up-to-date on what's happening.

In the end, smart home appliances could play an important part in strengthening home security in case of nuclear attack. They could provide immediate information, allow remote monitoring, regulate all aspects of your house, and aid in communications with family members as well as emergency aid. Owners of homes should look into adding smart devices to the plans for preparing to increase security.

www.ingramcontent.com/pod-product-compliance
Lightning Source LLC
Chambersburg PA
CBHW071337120626
46546CB00002B/599